# Women & Diabetes
## 2nd Edition

## Staying Healthy in Body, Mind, and Spirit

Skyline Medical Office
5125 Skyline Rd. S.
Salem, OR   97306

Laurinda M. Poirier, MPH, RN, CDE
Katharine M. Coburn, MPH

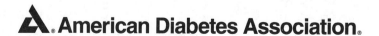
American Diabetes Association.

| | |
|---|---|
| *Book Acquisitions* | Robert J. Anthony |
| *Editor* | Sherrye L. Landrum |
| *Production Director* | Carolyn R. Segree |
| *Production Manager* | Peggy M. Rote |
| *Composition* | Circle Graphics, Inc. |
| *Cover Design* | Wickham & Associates, Inc., and KSA Group |
| *Printer* | Transcontinental Printing |

Printed in Canada
1 3 5 7 9 10 8 6 4 2

The suggestions and information contained in this publication are generally consistent with the *Clinical Practice Recommendations* and other policies of the American Diabetes Association, but they do not represent the policy or position of the Association or any of its boards or committees. Reasonable steps have been taken to ensure the accuracy of the information presented. However, the American Diabetes Association cannot ensure the safety or efficacy of any product or service described in this publication. Individuals are advised to consult a physician or other appropriate health care professional before undertaking any diet or exercise program or taking any medication referred to in this publication. Professionals must use and apply their own professional judgment, experience, and training and should not rely solely on the information contained in this publication before prescribing any diet, exercise, or medication. The American Diabetes Association—its officers, directors, employees, volunteers, and members—assumes no responsibility or liability for personal or other injury, loss, or damage that may result from the suggestions or information in this publication.

∞ The paper in this publication meets the requirements of the ANSI Standard Z39.48-1992 (permanence of paper).

ADA titles may be purchased for business or promotional use or for special sales. For information, please write to Lee Romano Sequeira, Special Sales & Promotions, at the address below.

American Diabetes Association
1701 North Beauregard Street
Alexandria, Virginia 22311

**Library of Congress Cataloging-in-Publication Data**
Poirier, Laurinda M., 1960–
    Women and diabetes: staying healthy in body, mind, and spirit / by
Laurinda M. Poirier and Katharine M. Coburn. — 2nd ed.
      p.    cm.
    Prev. ed. published with subtitle: Life planning for health and wellness.
    Includes index.
    ISBN 1-58040-058-2 (pbk. : alk. paper)
    1. Diabetes in women—Popular works.   2. Women—
Health and hygiene.   I. Coburn, Katharine M., 1962–    II. Title.

RC660.4 .P65 2000
616.4'62'0082—dc21
                00-38104

*In* memory of my sister, Leetha Poirier Trainer, whose life experiences and challenges continue to feed my passion for helping women to find their voices.

*To* my family, Jeanne and Donald, Loren, Lynnea, Luann, and Lyle, for their strength and inspiration.

*To* Lindsa, Deanna, Denise, Donna, Jan, and Katie for shared lessons and wisdom.

—*LMP*


*To* my mother, Lucie McKee, for sharing the poetry of daily life.

*To* my husband, Kevin Coburn, and our sons, Donald and Miles, for their love and support.

—*KMC*

# Struggle

*A man found a cocoon of the Emperor moth and
took it home to watch it emerge. One day a small
opening appeared, and for several hours the moth
struggled but couldn't seem to force its body past a
certain point.*

*Deciding something was wrong, the man
took scissors and snipped the remaining bit of
cocoon. The moth emerged easily, its body
large and swollen, the wings small and shriveled.*

*He expected that in a few hours the wings
would spread out in their natural beauty, but
they did not. Instead of developing into a creature
free to fly, the moth spent its life dragging around a
swollen body and shriveled wings.*

*The constricting cocoon and the struggle necessary
to pass through the tiny opening are God's way of
forcing fluid from the body into the wings. The
"merciful" snip was, in reality, cruel. Sometimes the
struggle is exactly what we need.*

—Jason Elias and Katherine Ketcham
*In the House of the Moon: Reclaiming
the Feminine Spirit of Healing*

# Contents

## Chapter 1

## Chapter 2

## Chapter 3

## Chapter 4

## Chapter 5

## Chapter 6

## Chapter 7

# Acknowledgments

*Our deepest appreciation goes to Dorothea F. Sims whose mentoring showed us that being well depends on the perspective to be gained in befriending diabetes and meeting life's challenges with optimism and grace.*

We express our gratitude to the women who personalized the messages in this book with their voices of reality: Deanna Kredenser, Margaret Lawlor, Lynn Fischhaber, and Dorothy DeMatteo.

A special thanks to Elizabeth C. Bashoff, MD, at the Joslin Diabetes Center, for her critiques along the way.

We thank Josie McKee and Allyson Coburn for their courageous ways of meeting their health challenges. They revealed to us how a woman mobilizes power when she chooses to respond to her challenges by growing through the experience. Their examples enrich so many lives.

A special thanks to Jennifer Potter, MD, staff physician at Beth Israel Deaconess Medical Center in Boston, instructor in Medicine at Harvard Medical School, for her assistance with the physical health chapter. Special thanks also to Ann E. Goebel-Fabbri, PhD, staff psychologist at Joslin Diabetes Clinic and instructor in Psychiatry at Harvard Medical School.

And finally (for her wisdom and support), we thank our editor, Sherrye Landrum, who made this possible.

# Woman's Ways: A Prelude

The most beautiful thing we can experience is the mysterious.

—Albert Einstein

In this book, you will be introduced to women who, at different times in their lives, made decisions, developed attitudes, or engaged in behaviors that did not serve them well. Their stories are about the dilemmas and choices that are involved in living as a woman with diabetes. It isn't important whether or not they take insulin or have the same type of diabetes that you do. Witness their internal struggles. How did their choices affect their self-care and feelings of well-being? What was it that helped them make the difference and pay attention to themselves?

These stories may make you realize things about yourself, what competes for your energy, and the impact of your choices. No matter what choices you made in the past, do not judge them. Look at your life with a new sense of hope. Learning to fit diabetes into your life as a partner, mother, sister, daughter, friend, or employee is an honorable challenge.

This book is for all women who live with the chronic disease, diabetes—young and old, type 1 and type 2, insulin users and non-insulin users. This is also for their loved ones who live and experience the struggles with them and for their health care providers who work beside them on their quest for wellness.

We view this book as a send-off, a bon voyage present. It does not make decisions for any of you but illustrates useful perspectives and strategies that may help you determine what you need, make decisions for your own wellness, and grow.

Life experiences as a woman with diabetes provide you with opportunities to learn more about your own wisdom, your unique gifts, and your powers. If allowed, diabetes can teach you that you are more than your body and more than a set of blood sugar levels. You are a whole and phenomenal woman. Having diabetes does not define you or your worth. Diabetes becomes a part of you, like the color of your eyes. It can become a teacher as well as a companion.

Diabetes forces you to grow and stretch in ways you never thought of—to learn a new language, new ways of thinking about your body, and new life strategies. Diabetes calls attention to the fact that you cannot take your body for granted. Your vulnerabilities become exposed as you experience the many unpredictable events in living with a chronic health condition.

The lessons are not always easy. For in living with a chronic health problem, you may encounter a sense of powerlessness, fear, or pain. Old wounds may surface in new ways, and insecurities or the pain of unrealized dreams may take you by surprise. Living through such challenges calls on your deepest wisdom. You'll need your intuition for healing, support, and guidance.

Life pushes and pulls. You are called to push back or to go with the flow. You have a choice. You can be locked in by your pain, losses, or disease. You can lose yourself, give up on your dreams and passions, and live in anger or resentment. Or you can embrace this part of you and do the work that can lead to an experience of joy and inner peace.

If you resist living with diabetes, you suffer. If you accept it as part of yourself, you can be happy. You will make mistakes because that is how we humans learn. When you forgive yourself and get fascinated by what is going on in your own life, you feel joy.

All women go through times when they do not honor themselves. Emotional and physical health suffers as a result. Over time, a woman may come to realize that her choices, attitudes, and behaviors are not helpful to her. By listening to the messages sent by her body, she will gain the insight to change and regain her honor. Her inner wisdom can guide her to a healthier state.

Some women realize this early in life, some later. Sometimes this awareness comes suddenly, causing a woman to make drastic changes in her self-care, relationships, or career choices. For other women, the realization is more gradual. However it happens, this insight does not remain constant. It has peaks and valleys. We get busy or forget, and need to become aware again. It is over time that we gain a deeper appreciation of what is best for ourselves.

We believe that living with diabetes is a journey—a physical, emotional, and spiritual journey. We hope that as you read this book you gain a sense of gentleness for yourself, a sense of humor to face life, and real energy to carry on. We invite you to participate actively in directing your life with diabetes instead of passively accepting what may happen. When you play an active role in your own life, you strengthen your sense of integrity. You come to know and then to honor what is right for you. You may not always be able to prevent a health problem or high and low blood sugars, but you can choose how you approach it and how you define your inner self. You do not have to lose sight of who you are because of it.

We write this book in honor of the woman with diabetes and for

her *story* and learning along the way,

her *joy* and *zest* for living,

her *desire* to feel whole, beautiful, and valued,

her *tears* that are the jewels of healing,

her *pain* and *fear* of the real and the imagined,

her *spirit* that is tender and giving, and

her *dreams* for a better tomorrow.

# Chapter 1

# My Own Reality

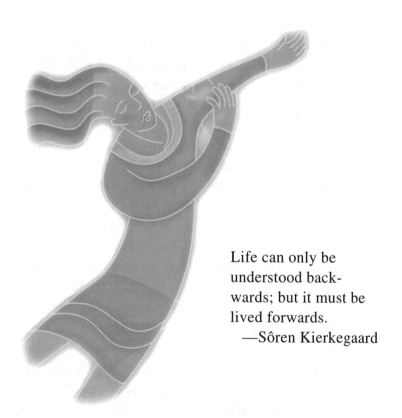

Life can only be
understood back-
wards; but it must be
lived forwards.
　　—Sôren Kierkegaard

*Anna was striking. At 72, she was radiant and beautiful despite the wrinkles, the dependency on a wheelchair for mobility, and even the recent loss of a grandchild. Her tenderness and comfort with herself radiated to others beyond the cloak of an aging body. She did not dwell on the fact that she was unable to keep up with the rest of the group nor that she needed help with some of her diabetes self-care tasks. Her focus was on living the moment, enjoying the view, and experiencing a new adventure. Her acceptance of herself enabled her to go beyond any external limitations and events imposed on her.*

Through Anna we see that it is possible to be well, despite having chronic health problems and disability. Wellness. Health. Whatever word you use, you need to develop an accepting relationship with yourself physically, emotionally, and spiritually. You can learn to live in harmony with your diabetes. Harmony comes from learning about your limits and your potential for change, as well as your physical and emotional needs. Diabetes is about confronting your vulnerability and your fears. It is also about hope. Living with diabetes calls you to make a promise to pay attention to yourself and to keep that promise.

We know that living with diabetes is not as simple as it sounds. It is tricky business learning how to take the right medication at the right time, eat the right amount of food, and exercise on schedule. You also need self-knowledge, communication skills, patience, and flexibility for adapting to unexpected events that can cause high and low blood sugars, which alter emotions and body functions. Whether you have type 1 or type 2, diabetes is with you every day. How you approach your diabetes physically, emotionally, and spiritually will affect the quality of your life, what you do, and how well you feel.

If you have not taken care of yourself or your diabetes in the past, don't waste energy now on regret or guilt. This will change nothing and is a poor investment of your precious time and energy. Acknowledge and respect the path that you have traveled this far and begin to explore how you can make a difference now. Consider the big picture and ask yourself: What do I want out of life as a woman who also happens to have diabetes? How do I want my life with diabetes to change? How do I need to adjust my approach to get there?

Most women want to do what is best for themselves, but knowing what is best and knowing how to do it are not always clear. It isn't easy to find the answer to questions such as how can I get into shape? what vitamins should I take? should I be on hormone replacement therapy or, what contraceptive pill is best for me? Discovering the answers that fit you requires time and trial and error. This can leave any woman feeling frustrated and overwhelmed. When you have diabetes, the normal dilemmas associated with being a woman can be magnified.

With diabetes there are no real milestones, so you may feel like you endlessly seek without ever arriving. To keep moving up and over the bumps in the road requires you to listen closely to your own body and to your inner voice. There are often no "right" answers, so you may have to try different approaches and make a few mistakes (experiments!) before you experience success. That is normal and to be expected.

Right now you have the opportunity to think about today and the future, to set some new life goals, and to explore ways to reach them. It's time to consider taking time for reflection and renewal. This is what teachers do when they go on sabbaticals and business people do during a retreat. It is the time to fuel your imagination, to be creative, and to have some fun, so that you can return to your life as a woman with diabetes in new ways that feel good to you and with new energies to keep you going.

In the midst of the turmoil of the day, we all need to take a moment, breathe deeply, and get clearer about what is important in our life and where to put our energy.

# Perfection: Is It Possible?

We all feel the pressure to be "Superwoman" at different points in our lives. Yet, it is never clear how Superwoman can do all that is expected of her. If you are trying to live up to images of the perfect woman or the perfect woman with diabetes, you will drive yourself crazy. No woman can orchestrate all of the factors that affect her health, the day's events, or her diabetes. Perfection is impossible, especially when you are managing a chronic disease. Striving to be perfect limits your ability to be present in the moment and can make you dissatisfied with your life. When your goals or expectations are unrealistic or inconsistent with who you are, you suffer. Your challenge is to accept that we are perfectly imperfect! We hope to help you feel better about letting go of any goals that require perfection and replacing them with more realistic expectations of what you can accomplish.

Do you ever find yourself comparing your body, your hair, or your accomplishments to those of other women and never feeling you are as good? On the surface, you can usually find (if you look hard enough) a woman you think is more beautiful, thinner, better dressed, more successful, or just luckier. Playing this comparison game drains your energy and diminishes your sense of self. The old wisdom of comparing yourself only to yourself is true. It is liberating to be happy about another woman's good fortune, while celebrating your own. This is a challenge all women have.

By whose standards do you judge yourself? Our society values women who are slim, successful, and wealthy. Do you try to mold yourself to fit these criteria, disregarding your own abilities, reality, and individuality? In the same way, do you just accept the health goals set by your diabetes care provider or do you participate in setting goals that are important to you? It is very easy to be tricked into defining your sense of worth by external measures like the numbers on the meter or the pounds lost. *Don't do it.* If you want to achieve wellness, you need to discard any images of so-called perfection and embrace your true self. These are good and powerful things to learn to do. This will improve not only your diabetes control, but the quality of your life.

Diabetes care is often demanding and gives few visible rewards. There will be highs and lows, undesired weight gain, and, sometimes, health problems. These things are not always within your control. If you believe that they are, you may unnecessarily burden yourself with guilt and shame. Focusing energy on those things that you can control and that add meaning to your life is much more productive. Now is the time to stop judging your actions as good or bad, successful or failure. This will be the beginning of your wisdom.

Women are, by nature, healers. You are one. You begin to heal when you listen to your own spirit and are true to yourself. Embrace your uniqueness! Look on any "mistakes" with a lighter heart because each one is simply an opportunity to learn. Treat yourself with respect and curiosity. You have the strength that you need to balance your vulnerabilities.

## My Partnership with Diabetes

To live in partnership with a chronic disease requires a habit of forgiveness—forgiving yourself for not being perfect, for making mistakes, for not giving it your best all of the time.

> *Mary says, "I have a hard time forgiving myself. I always think that I am never going to manage diabetes like I should. Other people can do it much better."*

No one can live perfectly with a chronic disease. Too many unpredictable events and circumstances affect glucose control, emotions, and body responses. Once you accept that, you give yourself the flexibility that you need to deal with the unexpected.

Each of us wants to be a whole woman whose life is full and balanced. To do that, we must recognize all the parts of ourselves and fit them together. In some ways, you might consider this as developing a relationship with yourself respecting both your light and dark sides. We all have them. As a woman with diabetes, however, you have an added responsibility to live in partnership with the light and dark aspects of your diabetes, too. How do you regard your diabetes? Is it a failure or a character flaw, something to be ashamed of or to hide? Do you think it detracts from your value as a woman? Is diabetes an enemy that drains you emotionally or physically, to fight and slay? Or is it a part of you that you accept and care for?

Consider how you would describe yourself to another person. Imagine that the circle below represents you, a whole person. Write in the words or qualities that describe you, your passions, likes, and strengths. Where would you place diabetes—inside or outside the circle? Take a moment to write the word *diabetes* where it fits best for you.

YOU

Did you say that you are a painter, a CEO, a mother, a martial artist, or a gardener? Did you note your passion for quilting, reading, or traveling? How did diabetes fit into the picture? Examine your circle again. How much energy do you give to each part of you? How much is your diabetes the focus of your life?

Let's examine how some other women have completed the circle. Which response rings true for you?

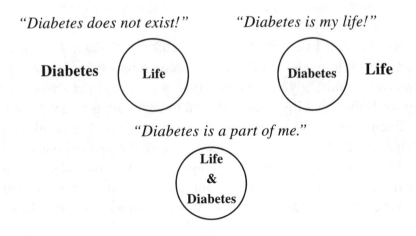

*"Diabetes does not exist!"*     *"Diabetes is my life!"*

**Diabetes**  Life          **Diabetes**  **Life**

*"Diabetes is a part of me."*

Life
&
**Diabetes**

## *Diabetes does not exist!*

*Susan wakes every morning, takes her medication, and puts her diabetes away for the rest of the day.*

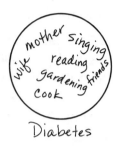

Diabetes

. For Susan, diabetes is placed outside of the circle. It is separate from her definition of self. She denies the presence of diabetes and lives her life making choices without regard to her health or to how her diabetes fits into the picture. She considers diabetes the enemy somehow, and she only deals with it when there is a problem. Women who share her point of view often make statements such as "I don't have time for diabetes. I will not let it control me. It will not get in the way." Words like fight, flaw, anger, fear, and resentment reflect their attitudes and emotions.

**Let's consider what happens when Susan treats her diabetes as separate from herself or as something bad.** Refusing to acknowledge the importance of diabetes can lead to poor diabetes control, which puts Susan at risk for other health problems. She may experience many low blood sugars that spoil her daily plans or high blood sugars that make her feel sluggish and ill. Susan may be putting herself at risk for diabetes complications such as eye disease or nerve damage.

When Susan denies her diabetes, she is not paying attention to her body nor is she respecting her own needs. For some women, having diabetes is like a barometer. The high and low blood sugars can teach you to look for something that is wrong. For example, Susan may be getting an infection or she may be under more stress than she realizes, and these conditions are reflected in her unexplained high blood sugars. Her blood sugar can offer her clues to help her stay in good health.

When Susan refuses to do diabetes tasks or approaches them with resentment, she is feeding herself negative and unhealthy messages.

Over time this dissatisfaction with the diabetes part of herself will create "dis" ease and imbalance. Denial builds stress and takes energy to maintain. In a sense, Susan is pretending that her diabetes does not exist.

**Why do women like Susan regard the diabetes part of themselves so negatively?** Having diabetes makes her feel different. She feels that she is not accepted by her peers, family, or society. It is difficult for people without diabetes to understand why she must eat a certain way or do special things for herself. High and low blood sugars complicate things even further. Other people may look at the strong emotions that accompany swings in blood sugar, like anger or crying, as exaggerated or just trying to get attention. They may not understand the issues behind those emotions. Other women may feel uncomfortable around her because her vulnerability can bring up fears of their own.

It is often difficult to take time from group activities to treat a low blood sugar or to recover from it. Susan may feel the need to overcompensate for the fact that diabetes got in the way, or she may feel ashamed. Considering this very common scenario, it is no surprise that Susan regards her diabetes as something bad and unwanted!

It is never comfortable exposing our sensitive side, weakness, or needs to others. Especially if these other people are critical of us or do not know us very well. We all want to be strong and perceived as well put together. By our own standards (or society's), we often feel that we should keep quiet about our own needs. Society seems to have little patience for people who are different or who focus attention on themselves. This may make it even more difficult for you to pay attention to your diabetes or any health need.

## *Diabetes is my life!*

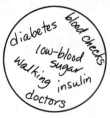

*Emma, who has type 2 diabetes, often refuses to join her friends at the bridge*

*club in order to be home to check her blood sugar and eat her meal on time.*

*Jennifer, with type 1 diabetes, works out every day after work, refuses to eat out with friends for fear of having to eat foods not on her meal plan, and checks her blood sugar five to ten times a day with the hopes of keeping them between 70–130 mg/dl. She is skeptical of dating because she feels that a prospective partner will think diabetes is a burden.*

Women like Emma and Jennifer define everything they do or are capable of doing by their diabetes. Diabetes is the major focus of their existence. Developing or creating healthy relationships with others, going to social functions, taking a job, having children, and even accepting spontaneous invitations are all limited by diabetes. Emma and Jennifer spend all their energy thinking about what to eat, how and when to exercise, and looking out for the next hypoglycemic episode.

Emma is paralyzed by fear. Getting together with friends would potentially expose her to situations that she does not feel she has control over such as foods that may cause blood sugars to go too high. Even more disturbing is the potential of having to face questions or suggestions from her friends about how she should deal with her diabetes.

Jennifer's sense of worth is defined by whether or not her blood sugars are within target. When they are not, she is miserable. She exercises more, eats less, and checks her blood sugar more often. Diabetes has become her life. Her life is not balanced; it is not full.

In both cases, Emma and Jennifer carry diabetes on their shoulders as a burden that controls their life. The special moments of the day, the miracles, the lessons, slip by them while they are focusing on their diabetes.

**How do women get into this trap?** Diabetes is complex. Keeping track of blood sugar levels, making treatment decisions, and responding to high and low blood sugars can easily consume your energy! You could spend a great deal of time trying to figure out why your blood sugar fluctuates and dealing with the emotional baggage like frustration or guilt that comes with the high or low blood sugars. It seems to be easier to turn down the invitation for dinner or let that new relationship go away than to deal with the fluctuations in blood sugar.

Motivated to be healthy by fear of complications, Emma and Jennifer try every moment of the day to achieve their health goals. Perhaps they have not learned how changes in food, activity, hormone levels, medications, or hectic schedules can affect their blood sugar, so they are constantly feeling guilty when blood sugars are outside of range. Trying to figure out each and every number is truly impossible.

It would help them to know that approximately 20–30% of blood sugar values can never be explained. In addition, they might benefit from knowing how to adjust their treatment approach so they could make changes in their schedules. When they learn how to change the amount of food or medication, they can feel free to enjoy events more fully.

It is not surprising that Emma's and Jennifer's lives are dominated by diabetes. Diabetes research and health care providers tell us to focus on blood sugars. This is because an important national study proved that keeping blood sugars as close to normal as possible reduces your risk for developing complications! Emma's and Jennifer's doctor fuels their unhealthy preoccupation with blood sugar levels by focusing on them. Because of limited time for routine office visits, health care providers may only have time to focus on blood sugar levels or other treatment goals. This leaves all the other ways to measure success unexplained and unexplored.

Even though your provider may not have the time to ask about how you are challenged emotionally or physically by diabetes, it is an important aspect of your self-care. It is ultimately your responsibility to seek out other people to support and to help you. Learning about your own body, your diabetes, and what affects you will help you keep diabetes in a balanced perspective. We give you some guidelines for working with your health care providers in chapter 4.

**What about you?**

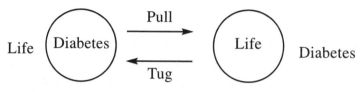

Many women find themselves going back and forth between two ways of relating to their diabetes. At one point it dominates their life; at another, it is ignored. This is normal. Expect it. However, if you get stuck in one of these ways of relating to your diabetes for long periods of time, you're out of balance and will face unhealthy emotional and physical consequences.

Now, let's consider how diabetes or any chronic health problem can become a part of your life. It is possible to learn how to pay attention to your diabetes and still keep it in a healthy balance with the rest of your life. Diabetes can be simply one aspect of your life that requires periodic attention and work.

Imagine the circle again with your diabetes in a positive light.

## *Diabetes is part of me!*

*B*renda *is a mom and a grandmother, with a part-time job and a home to maintain. She takes diabetes pills twice a day and monitors her glucose levels one to three times a day. She has learned to count carbohydrates and to adjust her food intake to fit in hiking with her family, dining out with friends, and biking.*

*Rebecca, 32, manages her diabetes with an insulin pump. She is constantly making decisions and trying to avoid hypoglycemia. She is a waitress and graduate student. She works hard at including time for relaxation and cross country skiing.*

Brenda treats diabetes as a priority along with other activities that she cares about. Diabetes does not carry a good or bad label. It just is. When it needs attention, she provides it, without resentment. Because she respects that diabetes is a part of who she is, she accepts that it will periodically challenge her. Once the challenge has been addressed, she can refocus her energy on other aspects of her life, such as gardening, child care, or work. To develop this balanced attitude toward her diabetes has required work. She learned a lot about her own body and about diabetes. She reached out to her family for support and to her health care team for guidance. She allowed herself to enjoy more moments, and perhaps a lesson, in each day.

Rebecca works equally hard at keeping her diabetes in perspective. At times she finds herself resenting her diabetes because it makes life difficult. Her resentment, even though it is strong, often serves as fuel for learning and being persistent. With the help of a friend and her doctor, she has found ways to work the important things into her life while managing her blood sugars. She doesn't ignore her diabetes or pretend it isn't there. She accepts it as part of her reality, and she's pleased with her life.

## Perceptions and Expectations

Fairly early in life, we arrive at an idea about who we are, what we are capable of doing, and how we should live. Sometimes we shortchange ourselves by these definitions or ideas. Instead of guiding us, these images act like a cage, actually preventing us from changing and growing.

*Marlene has found a hidden ability and passion for long-distance biking. Two years ago, her image of herself was not as an athlete. This self-definition was based on her awkward experiences with baseball and basketball as a child. Letting go of this limited self-image, she participated in a short bike-a-thon and found she enjoyed it. With subsequent bike trips, her enjoyment grew, and she was willing to go longer distances. One day she realized that she did have athletic abilities. They were just different from her notion of what being "athletic" was. Now, she enjoys this newfound part of herself and has learned that she does not have to bike at a competitive level to express herself in new ways or to have fun.*

So often, women limit their choices and enjoyment because of preconceived ideas or past experiences. Marlene was limited by two ideas. The first was that because she was not good at sports, she was not good at any athletic activity. The second was that she had to be good enough to compete. Releasing herself from these expectations brought her newfound joy! How often do your perceptions about yourself, your diabetes, or your previous experiences limit your potential today?

## Feeding Your Soul

You often hear "we are what we eat." In reality we are what we feed ourselves on several levels: the physical, spiritual, emotional, and intellectual. How do you nourish and replenish these areas? What messages do you feed yourself? What messages do you accept from others? Physically, we replenish our stores by eating healthfully, exercising, and getting enough sleep. To feed our hearts and minds, we give ourselves nurturing messages, think beautiful thoughts, read about and learn new things, and seek encouragement from others. We take a moment to be still and enjoy.

Consider what types of internal messages you accept from yourself or from others. Is there a critic inside you, ready to cut you down, one that actually drains your energy and confidence? Is there a harsh voice or a judge inside you who doubts your abilities? Or do you have an inner coach and personal cheerleader? Do you hear a nurturing and encouraging voice that tells you to reach for your dreams? Is there one that comforts you through difficult times? Do you tell yourself how great you are, despite any blunders or hurdles? Here are some messages other women have heard. Which ones feel more supportive and comfortable?

> *I can't do that! It isn't good enough!*
> *I've tried everything!*
> *It is possible. One thing at a time. I can do it.*
> *It is OKAY to make mistakes.*

What you feel and believe about yourself colors every experience you have. A woman who feels good about herself is likely to be able to cope with the crises in life better than the woman who feeds on negative messages.

What you choose to feed your body physically, emotionally and spiritually can be like putting money in the bank. Every time you make a deposit in the bank, your account grows larger. The larger the account, the more you have to draw on during hard times. If you constantly feed yourself negative or discouraging thoughts, you will find it very difficult to achieve any sense of health and wellness, especially during the hard times. Is it time to put some positive deposits into your emotional and spiritual bank, so that you have many encouraging and healing messages to feed yourself?

## Language: The Power of Words

The words we use to describe diabetes and ourselves will influence our experience, too. Medical jargon can be limiting or negative. Even though many of these terms cannot be avoided, being aware of the word and phrases that we use can help us achieve and maintain healthy balance in our lives.

Consider the words you use to talk about diabetes. Reflect on how these words make you feel about yourself as a woman. Look at the phrases below and choose the one that reveals the woman you are. Who lives inside the external cloak you see in the mirror?

*I am a diabetic!*—No, that isn't right!
*I am a person with diabetes!*—Yes, but I am more!
*I am a woman who happens to have diabetes*—That's right but more!
*I am a woman who is in touch with myself*
  *because of diabetes!*—YEAH!

Consider using the phrase that provides you with a sense of freedom to experience and celebrate yourself in new ways. We hope that you will value the idea that you are not just a diabetic. You are a woman, a person who has diabetes, with your own set of dreams, hopes and desires, unique gifts, and talents.

> *While attending a workshop, Sara learned that she could build a sense of well-being simply by adding the word "honor" to her vocabulary. The trainer in the course used words like honor when talking about a woman's body. Honor. The word alone is sweet, light, and respectful. That word had great impact on how Sara began to think about and care for her own body. She had been used to pushing herself day in and day out until exhaustion forced her to take refuge in sleep. Without meaning to, she had abused her body, taken it for granted, and responded to it only when it was completely exhausted. She had experienced many highs and lows. She did not feel vibrant and energetic. But in the workshop she learned that she should honor her body. When she realized that this is the only body she has and the vehicle that moves her along the journey of life, she embraced the value*

*of treating it better. After the workshop, she was more mindful about the types of food she fed her body, the amount of rest she had, and the ways she connected with her body.*

Words help give meaning to our experiences. This meaning feeds our beliefs and behavior. By including the word honor when speaking or thinking of herself, Sara began to feel better physically and emotionally.

## Reshaping Your Outlook

What does it take to regard diabetes as a healthy part of yourself? Honesty. Respect. Courage.

### *Honesty*
- about who you are
- about how you treat and take care of yourself
- about the choices you make
- about what you take for granted and what you ignore

### *Respect*
- for your individuality
- for the fact that all people make mistakes
- for the need to change your approach and attitude

### *Courage*
- to keep looking for truths
- to change
- to face our demons and release fears

How does having diabetes affect you? You experience emotions or physical feelings because of fluctuations in blood sugars that women without diabetes do not. All women feel, at some time, fatigued, irritable, lethargic, or overwhelmed. With diabetes, these feelings may be exaggerated and intense. Your ability to rebound may be a little slower. It isn't uncommon for women to deny that there is a problem and that their body requires more time to balance itself. Being aware of this will help you give yourself the time you need before you get overwhelmed.

Having diabetes does not make you better or worse than anyone else. It just is part of you. Diabetes is an issue of blood sugars and how food is used by the body. It does not define your value or worth. It is one of the challenges gifted to you. Your responsibility is to accept and to use what diabetes teaches you about yourself.

Do you have a golden opportunity to develop a healthy relationship with your diabetes? Your diabetes is there for you to respect—not to resign to—and to acknowledge it. It needs your attention. In this book, we explore how you can strengthen your relationship with yourself and with your diabetes. It is possible for all of us to get better at listening to our body's needs and developing the self-care skills that we need.

## Chapter 2

# Juggling Multiple Roles

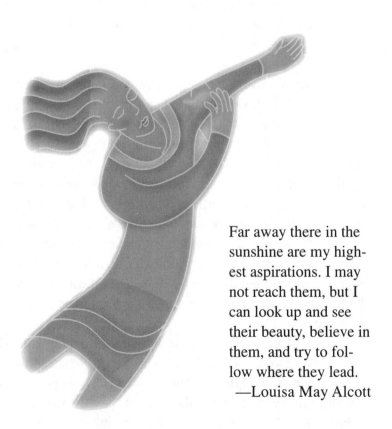

Far away there in the
sunshine are my high-
est aspirations. I may
not reach them, but I
can look up and see
their beauty, believe in
them, and try to fol-
low where they lead.
—Louisa May Alcott

*Joanie is a woman with diabetes, who works hard to keep her blood sugar level in target range. Lately she is distressed because only a few measurements have been within 80–150 mg/dl. She is frustrated and unhappy with the results. Feelings of failure and frustration begin to engulf her.*

*So what is going on? Sometimes, despite the best intentions and efforts, things get in the way of our plans. For instance, over the last two weeks, Joanie has had additional pressures from work and a sick loved one to care for, which has added stress and leaves no time to follow her activity program and little time for herself. She is a woman juggling many demands on her time and energy. It isn't surprising that her diabetes control is less than ideal.*

Have you ever wondered why you feel exhausted at the end of the day? Or why blood sugar levels do not cooperate with even the best-laid plans? There are good reasons why achieving glucose control, achieving your goals for the day, and maintaining wellness are daily challenges. As a woman, you may juggle demands from work and home, along with addressing personal needs and the health care demons of diabetes. As a woman with diabetes, you also have to integrate all these demands with the daily responsibilities of managing diabetes. Unexpected events and requests from others may periodically distract you from attending to your self-care needs. If left unchecked, these demands can easily consume your energy, leaving you drained and falling short of your life goals.

To manage your life and your diabetes with integrity and a sense of self-worth you need to develop an ability to set limits (say no), to place yourself high on your list of priorities (say yes), and to use support systems (friends, family, health providers, support groups, etc.). How aware are you of the many demands placed on you? How prepared are you to deal with those demands? Through the activities in this chapter, you have the opportunity to see what you do on a daily basis and what you need to do to create more balance in your life. Keep a sense of humor as you as you explore what your life is really about and see how expectations of perfection set you up for disappointment and frustration.

Once you know what is asked of you, you can determine what skills, behaviors, and attitudes you need for dealing with the demands of being, first a woman and, then a woman with diabetes. It takes a lot of know-how. The next step is to commit to taking action. It is important to use the skills and adopt the positive attitudes and behaviors that serve you best. This is a challenging task. You may need to call on your inner "coach," that wiser self, to get rid of negative thoughts that sabotage your efforts. Likewise, you might want to ask for help from other coaches, those people who can push you when you need to be pushed or guide you when you need additional insight.

Life presents many challenges. Are you choosing the path you're following? Or are you being pulled here and there by life events and other demands? Are you developing your own signature style of being? The stories in this chapter may help you become more aware of the choices you've already made and reveal some other choices that you can make for yourself.

## Appreciate All of What You Do

Consider what is involved in your day-to-day life as a woman with diabetes, a woman juggling multiple roles and demands. You might discover that you are communicating, learning, negotiating, making decisions, taking time out for play and rest, and connecting with loved ones. In addition to cooking, cleaning, and shopping, you might find yourself periodically taking time out to check blood sugars, take medication, or treat a low blood sugar. While fulfilling your duties in the work force or tending to the home, you might need to fit time in to care for children or an aging parent.

Living with any chronic condition also requires working with family, friends, and health care providers to develop or follow strategies for managing all of your health care needs. In reality, it is a balancing act between prioritizing your needs with those of others. Your challenge is to fit diabetes into your other lives—as a partner, mother, sister, and friend. Diabetes demands that you become a master juggler.

You need mental, physical, and technical skills to care for diabetes and other self-care needs while maintaining your home, family, and work life. Does any woman come fully equipped with all the skills and tools necessary? Nope. No one does. But you can learn new skills by paying attention to yourself and accepting a little help from the people with whom you share your life.

Take a moment to appreciate all that you do and contribute to yourself and to others. Reflect on the things that you do on a routine basis, outlining your responsibilities in all your roles, such as partner, mother, daughter, employee, boss, volunteer, athlete, student, teacher, artist, or friend. Write them in the box below. Then add to the list what you do to take care of your diabetes. The self-assessment lists at the end of this chapter can help you complete this inventory. You might be surprised at all that you are juggling!

---

### Routine Tasks

The things I need to do on a routine basis include

---

### Diabetes Tasks

The things I need to do to take care of my diabetes includes

---

How do these lists compare to each other? Are any of your responsibilities in competition with each other for your time and energy? Do you feel any one area is neglected? Being aware of these responsibilities as well as how much time you devote to them is important. Putting too much time in one area or too many things on your to-do list, can create imbalance and a sense of "dis"ease. If you divide yourself up too much, you lose focus and effectiveness. Saying yes to too many of the roles that you juggle will result in many balls hitting you all at one time. Not saying no when you need to, keeps you away from yourself, so you lose awareness and time that you need to take care of your emotions, physical needs, or desires. Eventually, this takes its toll. Your emotional and physical health suffer. Can you afford that?

Let's look at the demands that compete with Margot's and Betty's abilities to take care of themselves.

*Margot is a single woman. Her job as a graphic artist often requires her to work late and occasionally on weekends. Because she does not rely financially on someone else, she feels pressure to work in a job that will provide her with a certain income and good retirement benefits. She invests a great deal of time going to seminars and taking classes to enhance her career opportunities. Margot spends her free time helping her sisters take care of her nieces and nephews. She also puts energy into developing and maintaining friendships. Friends operate as family in many situations for support, guidance, and laughter. In between her class, work, and social schedule, Margot finds it hard to fit in time to work out and take care of her diabetes. Her blood sugar levels bounce all over, ranging from 40 to 320 mg/dl. At times, she feels anxious and overwhelmed with it all.*

*Betty is a wife, a mother of two grown children, and a teacher at the junior high school. She shares the financial and household responsibilities with her husband. She is often tired and drained after dealing with her students. Her days are long, as she grades papers, helps troubled students, and prepares for classes. She is an active member of her church community and joins in running craft fairs and other fundraisers. She and her husband enjoy round-dancing and visiting with their children. She works not only for her own satisfaction and personal growth but also to help support her children in college and pay for the added expense of diabetes supplies. She struggles with her weight, and her blood sugars are often higher than desired. She often feels defeated and tired.*

Both Margot and Betty work hard to balance all the demands on their time. They know that it is important to take time out for their health, but sometimes, it is difficult. Their unconscious desire is to do everything well. They strive to keep their blood levels less than 150 mg/dl most of the time, keep their weight stable, and take care of daily chores, work demands, and family needs without a mistake. No wonder they feel overwhelmed or fatigued!

How realistic are Margot's and Betty's expectations of themselves? How much are you like them, trying to be Superwoman and do everything well? How often do you find yourself having to do everything alone or assuming responsibilities for too many things? Is there an opportunity in your life to share the load with another person or to eliminate a few commitments?

## Making You a Priority

Where are *you* on the list of priorities? Are you like many other women who put their needs last? What happens when you do that? When a woman fails to tend to her own needs, she begins to wither away physically and spiritually. Resentment replaces joy. Depletion replaces energy. Living with diabetes, or any health problem, demands that you make yourself a priority. It requires you to take the time to listen to your body and to respond to it in a way that is healthful. Otherwise high and low blood sugars, fatigue or illness will overcome you and zap your energy. And when you don't feel well, you can't get much of anything done or enjoy anything you do.

In our society it is considered admirable for a woman to sacrifice herself and minister to the needs of others. This can make it difficult and uncomfortable for you to say no to others, so you can do something for yourself. In some cases, a woman may feel selfish or guilty or feel badly that she is disappointing someone. It may also be hard to say no when you know you are capable. Yet, if a woman is to achieve wellness, it is critical for her to learn how to gently balance her needs with those of others. Learning to balance "yes" with "no" is one of the most important life skills a woman can develop.

We hope that at this moment, you are congratulating yourself on all you do! Call a friend or loved one and celebrate this new awareness. Your responsibilities help you learn more about your abilities, your strengths, and your potential to grow. They also allow you to confront the reality that you are not superwoman. No one is.

The issues in this chapter were not raised to provide you with an excuse for uncontrolled blood sugars or not paying attention to yourself. Quite the opposite, we hope that you will pay more attention to yourself and your diabetes care, so that you can enjoy a more fulfilling life. We present these issues to raise your awareness of the many roles you fulfill and of the demands that may make it difficult for you to achieve health goals. We hope that you can appreciate the importance in balancing your needs with those of others. Responding to the push and pull of daily life without such balance can interfere with the quality of your life. If you lose sight of yourself, things can spiral out of control leading to decreased emotional health, feeling negative, decreased attention to self, and ultimately to poor physical health. You must first value who you are before you feel moved to take care of yourself.

## Putting It into Perspective

Let's put this into perspective. The schedule you keep for blood glucose control may not coincide with your family activities, your work demands, and your social life. As one woman described it, diabetes consists of a 7-day work week with no vacations or weekends! You are expected to manage your diabetes in an environment that can be unpredictable and filled with other people's suggestions of what to do.

Examine the nature of your life with diabetes—the physical demands, the emotional challenges, the support systems (or lack of them). Identify what is chaotic and stressful, and what is productive and supportive. Think about who is there to listen and to help you in your quest for health and wellness. Be gentle as you unveil the elements of your world. Be honest about what or who depletes your energy.

Explore ways to build your self-esteem and confidence, to strengthen your ability to be an advocate for yourself, and to enhance your ability to communicate. Notice who or what recharges and supports you. If the demands seem too great or the environment is harsh, consider reaching out for the support and guidance that you need to protect and nourish you.

Over time you may find that your skills are not enough to reach your current goal or to meet the demands facing you. Your body will change, resulting in changes in blood sugar levels, medication needs, and overall blood glucose control. To meet these new demands, you may need to fine tune your diabetes skills, learn new ones, or develop a different approach to the situation. A diabetes-care provider can help you adjust your treatment program to dine out without experiencing hypoglycemia or help you design a flexible daily schedule for a more relaxed lifestyle. Begin to think about what new skills you need to achieve your lifetime and blood glucose goals. Ideas for enhancing your skills and ability to manage life with diabetes are explored in greater detail in the chapters that follow.

## Feedback

As human beings we thrive on receiving feedback about where we stand, how well we are doing and where we need to improve.

Some of the feedback comes from within and some from external sources. Receiving feedback about how well you are doing and where you can improve gives you the insight to create balance in your life. Creating healthy feedback mechanisms can help you avoid losing sight of yourself and redirect you when you are straying too far from your true interests.

Receiving words of thanks for the little gesture given, for putting a meal together at the end of a hectic day, or pulling a project together at work reinforces our knowing that we are on the right path. Words of support and encouragement from loved ones can provide feedback that motivates us to keep on track or face the difficult times. Comments like the following ones can provide us with the acknowledgment that what we do makes a difference.

*I appreciate how hard you are working at losing weight.*
*Keep up the good work. I see you trying. I believe in you.*
*I appreciate all that you do.*
*You manage so many things that other people don't even think*
*of ever doing.*

Sometimes, you need to ask for feedback, letting people know what it is that you need from them. What gestures do you want to receive? It is up to you to determine what you want to hear or receive from others and then to share that insight with them. Otherwise, it is unfair to expect that they will read your mind and know how to meet your unspoken need.

*After 18 years of marriage, Catherine learned that if*
*she wanted to receive flowers for her birthday, she*
*needed to tell her husband that that would make her*
*feel good.*

Feedback about your worth and value also comes from inside you. What feedback messages do you give yourself? Is the inner critic always reminding you about your faults or misgivings? Or is the inner mother available to calm, soothe, and support you as you face the unpredictable events of the day? Learning to be positive with yourself is important (especially when you do not receive this feedback from others). You will learn more about this in chapter 7.

Your monitoring results, such as glycohemoglobin levels, your body weight, cholesterol level, and the blood glucose checks you do at home help you evaluate the effectiveness of the choices you make or the plan that you follow. Your energy levels, the tone of your muscles, and the ability to walk longer today than you did last week is also physical feedback telling you about your progress. How well do you listen to your body? Are you tuned into the message that you hear? Is your body telling you that things need to be different?

Are you clear about what feedback you need and how you will measure your own accomplishments? What standards are you using? Keep in mind our discussion about using realistic and fair standards to compare yourself to.

## Taking Time to Recharge

We have all heard the old saying, "take time to smell the roses." How often do you stop to appreciate the experiences you have every day—the accomplishments, the lessons, and the miracles? The fast pace of today's world easily draws us into overdrive and fatigue. We often try to overcome even the natural limitations of time and energy. We fill our lives with enough for a 40-hour day!

Living in this way for any length of time leaves us depleted and out of touch with ourselves and our bodies. A critical but often unexplored aspect of life with a chronic health problem is creating time off from all the responsibilities, time to recharge and replenish our energy. This is truly important for you. Energy is stored in physical, emotional, and spiritual banks. You draw on these energy accounts to deal with the daily tasks that include diabetes. These are also the stores that help you through those crises with diabetes that call for a great deal of energy. When your resources are limited or depleted, you can't cope as well. It is easy to misinterpret events and react out of hurt or fatigue instead of responding to the actual event with calm consciousness.

Consider taking time out from some of your day-to-day responsibilities or diabetes tasks. Now is the time to explore how to do this and protect your greatest investment—yourself. It is true that you are unable to put diabetes on the shelf on Thursday and come back to it on Monday. But you can unload some of your responsibilities by asking a loved one to check your blood sugars and be responsible for your medication schedule. Or you might negotiate with someone else to do the cooking, cleaning, or shopping for a few days. Step out of the daily grind to give yourself something that makes your soul smile—like a special phone call, a hot bath, or a snuggle.

*Take time off!*
*Replenish your stores!*
*You are worth it!*

## Transitions

Consider again your diabetes responsibilities with greater appreciation for the day-to-day tasks that achieve wellness. When you realize all the demands on your time, you can appreciate why it is so important to nurture and take care of yourself. When you do, you are more resilient and able to be present for the other people in your life over the long run.

This is the time to take stock and commit to yourself. Direct some of your caring energy inward. You may need help to do this. Make yourself a priority. The key is to listen and respond to the wisdom of your own body. Managing life as a woman with diabetes provides you with a powerful opportunity to discover more about your own wonderful qualities and to express yourself in new ways. Take a moment now to give yourself a pat on the back, a hug, and words of appreciation. You are a remarkable woman!

## Assessing My Roles and Responsibilities
## as a Woman with Diabetes

This checklist outlines typical roles and responsibilities of women who live with diabetes. To help you appreciate all that you do, consider going through this list and checking off what you are responsible for. Are there other roles you play? Share your insights with loved ones who can celebrate all that you do.

### General Self-Care

○ Rest when you need to. If you are tired, stop and give your body a break.

○ Practice relaxation techniques.

○ Get plenty of sleep.

○ Exercise regularly.

○ Drink 6–8 cups of caffeine-free, alcohol-free, sugar-free fluids (water) each day.

○ Lubricate your skin if it is dry.

○ Seek out emotional assistance if life is overwhelming and if you are feeling depressed.

○ Determine what your needs are and seek ways to meet them.

○ Prioritize your needs and the needs of others. Determine how to balance them. Share the tasks.

○ Respect your body and the unique health need that is has.

○ Accept other people's help.

○ Engage in activities that allow you to be creative; do things you enjoy.

### Home Care (May or may not be shared with a spouse or roommate.)

○ Do the shopping and cooking.

○ Do the cleaning and laundry.

○ Do maintenance and home repair.

○ Keep the lawn mowed, the garden tended.
○ Empty the garbage routinely.

**Other People Care**
*Child care*
○ Feed and clothe the family.
○ Keep watch and respond to their ongoing developmental and health care needs.
○ Care for their emotional needs. Comfort them when sad or scared. Celebrate their joys. Provide discipline as needed.
○ Bathe them and tuck them in.
○ Get them off to school or day care on time and safely.
○ Help them off to college or transition into adult hood.
○ Organize social outings, all the way from preparing to cleaning up and putting away.
○ Function as the diplomat and mediator in the family, seeking to keep peace between all family members and resolve the small wars that seem to present themselves.
○ Serve as the confidant, advisor, and informer, always prepared to allow your ideas to be discarded or argued with.
○ Baby-sit and care for grandchildren when and if needed.

*Parent care*
○ Bring parent to doctor appointments and help address the effects of current illnesses.
○ Develop strategies to ensure safety and comfort.
○ Do the cooking, cleaning, and home repairs as needed.
○ Assist with financial management and personal care as needed.
○ Share creative activities.

*Relationships*
○ Respond to the needs and desires of your spouse or partner.
○ Communicate needs and desires clearly.

## Other People Care (continued)

○ Negotiate conflicts smoothly.

○ Give time to the relationship even when it means delaying going to bed at the end of an exhausting day.

○ Do something special for that extra-special somebody in your life.

○ Receive gifts, suggestions, and even criticism gracefully. Figure out what is important to you so you can learn about yourself.

○ Entertain and connect with friends.

○ Be open to asking for support and letting others support your efforts.

○ Work well as a team.

## Diabetes Self-Care

○ Choose what and when to eat.

○ Monitor blood sugar as often as you and your health care provider decide is best.

○ Enjoy some physical activity every day.

○ Respond to blood sugar levels that are outside of desired range.

○ Check your feet daily, washing and lubricating them as needed.

○ Take your medication in the right amount, at the right time, and using the right technique.

○ If you take insulin, adjust the dose after careful consideration of the factors that can cause your blood sugar to go too high or low.

○ See a dietitian or nurse educator for a review and fine-tuning your skills.

○ See your doctor routinely, 2–4 times a year.

○ Together with your providers determine goals for diabetes.

○ Work out the small steps it will take to reach your goal.

○ Apply the diabetes care principles that you learn.

○ Watch to see how your choices and behaviors affect glucose control and overall health.

### Diabetes Self-Care (continued)

○ Tell your provider what parts of the plan are difficult or not working for you.

○ Determine what your needs are and communicate them. Ask for help when you are tired or unable to pay attention to your needs.

○ Think through the steps you need to take to prevent and to treat high and low blood sugars.

○ Work as THE captain of the team.

### Risk Factor Reduction

○ If you smoke, stop. Or look into smoking cessation programs.

○ If you have high blood pressure, high cholesterol, or high triglycerides, follow a meal plan and take prescribed medications to bring levels into the desired range.

○ If you are overweight, improve your eating and activity habits to support your efforts in losing or preventing further gain.

**Employment** (For those who also work outside the home)

○ Complete projects and responsibilities as requested.

○ Maintain professionalism at all times.

○ Conduct yourself in a customer-friendly manner.

○ Do not let home and social life interfere with work.

○ Be efficient and courteous.

○ Accommodate your job assignments while simultaneously taking care of the household and family.

○ Minimize frequency and impact of highs and lows in the work setting.

# Chapter 3

# Moving Along Your Own Path

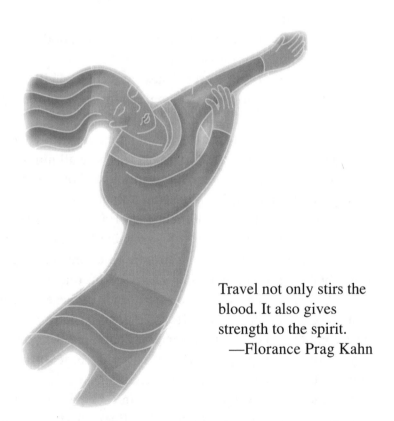

Travel not only stirs the
blood. It also gives
strength to the spirit.
　—Florance Prag Kahn

M oving through life as a woman with diabetes exposes you to interesting experiences and challenging adventures. How comfortable you are in this journey depends on what having diabetes means to you, your life experiences, and the way you approach living. Comfort comes from having a positive outlook, reasonable expectations, and adequate life experience to guide you. A new experience is less comfortable than one you have had often. Your degree of comfort is also dependent on your attitude toward it. To move with ease and grace you need to be able to gather support and information, so that you know generally what to expect and allow yourself enough time to get the experience. This chapter helps you think about where you are and what to expect on the three different paths you take as a woman with diabetes.

1. **Diabetes:** from being newly diagnosed to incorporating diabetes into your identity.
2. **Womanhood:** from birth through childhood, adolescence, adulthood, and into maturity.
3. **Wellness:** from treating illness and coping with disability to a wider definition of personal health and well-being.

If you are like most women, you do not deal with your diabetes, life challenges, and health separately. They're all jumbled up. You will not move through your life journey without retracing steps, taking detours, and hitting impasses. Smooth travel in one area fosters smoother travel on another. Sometimes managing the challenges of your life (diabetes, life, and health) seems effortless. At other times, nothing is easy. You may find yourself struggling to find your way as the demands of your life, diabetes, and health clash. Understanding where you are in each of these areas will give you insight into what new information, skill, perspective, or support you need to deal with a specific challenge. As you would on any journey, you progress as you experience, learn from it, and become motivated to take on new challenges.

First, let's discover where you are in each part of your journey. This helps you appreciate how each influences you. Second, we'll weave the three pathways of your life journey together to see how they interact to shape your life experience as a woman with diabetes. We hope that along the way you will identify a few things in your life to pay special attention to and develop some strategies for setting and reaching your goals.

## Making Diabetes Part of Your Life

Accepting diabetes happens gradually and is a continual process. Integrating diabetes into your life does not mean that you're problem free but acknowledges the problems as just another part of who you are. Integrating a new part into yourself is cyclical in nature. As you come to terms with one aspect of having diabetes, you may then be ready to deal with another aspect and the acceptance process begins anew. For example, after learning how to follow a meal plan based on exchanges and measuring portion sizes as part of your eating habit, you may become frustrated that it doesn't allow you to be as flexible as you'd like. You have to learn a new method that allows you to match what you eat with your busy work schedule and caring for your children. Carbohydrate counting may be the best choice for you now, but the idea of having to read labels again makes you hesitate before trying this new approach. Once again you may find yourself dealing with the need to accept diabetes all over again.

There are two different faces of acceptance here. First, you accept diabetes as part of who you are. Second, you accept each of the things that you need to do to live with it. How you relate to yourself as a woman with diabetes is unique. You are the only one who understands what having diabetes is really like for you. However, the process of accepting diabetes does follow some predictable steps.

### *Moving in*

This initial step begins with diagnosis and involves "learning the ropes." You are a novice, a beginner. Through experimenting and learning from it, you will determine how to take on the new responsibilities given to you. You begin to realize what strengths, resources, and influence you can bring to the new challenge. It may all seem overwhelming. You might feel like a misfit. This is because it is so new, and you haven't gained any useful diabetes life experiences yet.

With no prior experience and little preparation, you are suddenly awarded a new position in life. And you must begin training promptly because it will soon become one of your major life responsibilities. Things move very quickly after diagnosis. Often, the newly diagnosed person is trained to be a walking encyclopedia of diabetes facts, without anyone ever considering how she will integrate the new demands into her personality, life skills, or competing demands.

Ideally you need diabetes education gradually over time because absorbing new information and integrating changes in your lifestyle takes time. You may feel overwhelmed by the health care team members who are telling you what to do. You'll probably go through some form of denial at this stage. It's normal whenever you have to adjust to an unexpected event. All of us resist change and cling to our familiar lifestyle, even if it doesn't work for us anymore.

Try to learn (or relearn) about diabetes in manageable chunks. At first you just need to know what to do each day to survive, later you can learn how your diabetes care can be modified to match your lifestyle. It is very important to share the details about your everyday lifestyle and schedule with your health care providers so you can work together to develop a diabetes care plan that fits. If it doesn't fit you, you won't wear it. You are the only one who knows what will work for you. This is an important responsibility. After "moving in" you are ready to take over leadership of your health care team. Your health care team should be working for you to fit the new demands of diabetes in with the rest of your life. When you clearly communicate your needs, resources, and challenges, you and your health care team can set realistic goals for you.

Over time you might find that one aspect of your lifestyle or your diabetes care no longer suits you. This will cause you some discomfort, forcing you to reexamine things, and possibly to make changes. Anytime there is a change, you begin again the cycle of accepting

# Diabetes Diagnosis Exercise

How old were you when you developed diabetes?

_____

What responsibilities did you have and how confident in meeting them were you?

_____

What financial challenges were you faced with?

_____

What was your first reaction to the diagnosis of diabetes?

_____

What was the reaction of close family and friends?

_____

What was your relationship like with your health care providers?

_____

Did you understand what was happening to your body and why?

_____

Were there people available to answer your questions and help you fit the demands of diabetes into your life?

_____

Were your initial needs taken care of?

_____

What lingering needs from your initial diagnosis are still unmet?

_____

your diabetes. You can return to this level no matter what your age as you experience changes in your life, health, and diabetes care.

Emily, a 45-year-old accountant and mother of three didn't experience negative feelings about diabetes until years after her diagnosis. Emily only now has recognized the emotions she felt when she had to make so many changes.

*When I was first diagnosed, I had just lost a young nephew in an accident, and my brother was diagnosed with cancer. When they told me that I had diabetes, I thought "no big deal." In comparison to what my family had to deal with, diabetes was manageable. At first, I thought of it as an inconvenience but felt confident that I could figure out what and when to eat, and take the medication the correct way. But now, things are different. I dealt with it better then than I do now. When I realized that diabetes was going to last forever and the early symptoms of complications appeared, I began to feel how much freedom I had lost. Recently, my doctor told me that my kidneys were spilling small amounts of protein. Yikes! I wanted to take care of it right then. Then the eye doctor told me that I had small dot hemorrhages in my eyes. I was, and still am, so frightened and angry that I have to deal with this.*

Emily has worked hard to take care of herself. At first she thought that meant she was not supposed to have problems. But, as we know, it isn't that easy and simple because the body is complex. Many factors contribute to physical health, some that Emily has no control over. Her efforts were of value however! Emily was able to prevent the problems from developing earlier because she did take care of herself. And she had them diagnosed early. This is the time when treatment is most effective. She and her health care provider can keep an eye on these problems and prevent them from getting worse. What lies ahead depends on the collaboration between her and her health care team. She can throw up her hands in despair or take a deep breath and keep taking one step at a time.

## Moving through

After recovering from the initial shock of being told you had diabetes, you began to form beliefs about why you developed the disease, who you are now, and what you will need to do differently. For example, many people think that eating too much sugar causes diabetes (but it doesn't). Many people believe that you can't ever eat sugar again if you have diabetes (but you can). These beliefs may be at the heart of your refusal to follow your meal plan now. You need to look at what you believe about diabetes to see whether those beliefs are limiting your growth. The information, support, and guidance you received at diagnosis helped shape your current beliefs, but you should evaluate them now and replace those that no longer serve you well.

This more settled phase happens as you gain experience, develop regular diabetes care habits, and learn how to cope with unplanned events. You reach a plateau, a level of comfort and familiarity. You may feel more confident. You know what to expect. Many people become bored with the routine and frustrated by the unpredictability of living with diabetes. The new demand—to maintain your commitment and interest—is actually far greater than the demands during the first stage when everything was new.

Lucy "learned the ropes" of taking care of her diabetes long ago. Doing these tasks is second nature to her, but the resistance to doing them comes back periodically. The spark of newness or excitement about coping with the challenges that diabetes brings is now gone. Becoming bored with the routine is predictable, but it is a problem that can interfere with anyone's commitment and level of motivation.

> *I get tired of it all the time. It is so monotonous and requires too much structure. Eat now, check blood sugar, take medication. I can't get away from the clock! Sometimes because of stress, hormones, hunger,*

*or fatigue, I don't feel like exercising. Sometimes I get sick of it all!*

*Taking care of my diabetes takes time. I have to think about what I am going to eat, figure what my dose should be, and take time to check my blood sugar. I get tired of these tasks and having to take time out of my day that I don't want to give up. I feel trapped!*

Time for renewal and rejuvenation may be just what Lucy needs. She wants and deserves a break. She can excuse herself from the dull routine and ask for help in sharing the tasks that are really tough. She can take a mental vacation and talk with her health care provider about new treatment strategies. She can also take a class on any topic that might juice up her life, and help her regain her enthusiasm. Seeking out the ear of a good friend may help.

Diabetes is no longer the "new kid on the block." As you get to know it better, its little quirks can be annoying and tiring. Complacency can be a problem, too. It is easy to want to go with the flow and lose sight of the importance diabetes brings to your life. That's when life events or body changes can shake things up and possibly demand that you renew your acceptance of diabetes again.

## *Moving along*

This phase of renewal involves more change. It occurs when you realize that your approach no longer matches your current situation and needs. It is from the work done in this phase that you identify new goals and expectations. You begin to see yourself in a new way. The challenge here is to take stock of where you are and to take charge of getting to where you want to be. You may have to seek new knowledge, heal emotional wounds, or revise treatment plans. This stage may come as a surprise, out of the blue. Life influences your diabetes. Diabetes influences your life. As the body changes, your diabetes may change too. As your diabetes changes, your body may change. During this period of time it is not uncommon for a woman to revisit many of the emotions she first experienced when diagnosed.

You may not always be thinking about your diabetes and for the most part, you feel like you accept it. Then, without warning, something happens (developing retinopathy, having a serious insulin reaction, being rejected by the man you love), that challenges this level of acceptance. Once again, you are faced with the need to spend time getting comfortable with your diabetes in order to move along.

Edie is 48 years old and has had type 1 diabetes for 11 years. She is single and maintains a career as a graphic artist. Work and social commitments keep her very busy. Her diabetes-care program involves taking three shots of insulin a day (regular and NPH at breakfast, regular at supper, and NPH at bedtime), checking blood sugar 1–4 times a day, and counting carbohydrates. She is committed to following an exercise program as a form of relaxation as well as for glucose management. This has not always been the case. Over the years, her ability and willingness to pay attention to her physical and emotional needs were overwhelmed by competing priorities and life events. Periodically situations arise that challenge her acceptance of her diabetes.

> *Traveling for my job is difficult. Occasionally I have to fly across time zones. This does such a number on my blood sugars, and I end up feeling horrible. I can't seem to manage my blood sugar levels as well as usual or exercise as often. And the food! I am either relying on airline food or eating in restaurants. Diabetes can be such a hassle. I asked to be reassigned to an intercontinental route and the demands of managing my blood sugars became much more manageable.*

It is hard to accept such a complicated challenge, especially when you didn't ask for or expect it. Yet, unless you reach a sense of wholeness as a woman who happens to have diabetes, your energy gets locked up in fighting or denying it, preventing you from fulfilling other needs.

## Where are you?

Let's take a minute to look at what living with diabetes means to you right now and how your experiences have shaped your attitude and behaviors related to having diabetes.

1. What is the most difficult part of having diabetes for you right now?
2. How did you resolve earlier challenges?
3. What about having diabetes do you ignore?
4. How has your attitude to having diabetes changed since the first year after being diagnosed?

Let's look at how two different women "moved in" with diabetes and are living with it.

Ellen, an energetic cat-lover was 5 years old when she was diagnosed with diabetes. She vividly remembers this and how she decided that having diabetes wasn't going to change her life.

*She remembers being in the hospital. She was overjoyed with all the attention she was getting. She especially remembers being in a cage-bed full of toys and being able to ask the nurse for juice whenever she wanted. Grape juice parties with the little boy in the next bed were fun. Ellen would reach through the bars and say "cheers" before gulping down her juice. She couldn't understand why her parents seemed so concerned. She understood that things were not okay when the nurse answered her request for another juice party with, "Ellen, you can't have grape juice anymore. You have diabetes." This was the first of many painful realizations and changes. But she was determined not to let anything wreck her parties. She replaced juice parties with swapping toys with the little boy. Taking shots and weighing food were part of the routine, like brushing her teeth. She quickly learned that if she did what "they" asked her to, she could do most of what she wanted to. This is still the way Ellen views having diabetes. She keeps diabetes in reasonable control and is able to lead her life as she pleases. She'll find a way to see the positive even when things are really bad. Ellen remarked, "Looking back, I think that because I have diabetes, I look harder for things to celebrate, take greater risks, and work harder to accomplish more than most people."*

Dorothy, a retired high school teacher, now 58, was diagnosed when she was 47. Her diagnosis was a blur. She hardly remembers when she first began to feel bad but remembers clearly realizing how much her daily routine would be forever changed by the diagnosis. She first became aware that something was wrong when she was on vacation, visiting her sister.

*She felt groggy and sick to her stomach. Her sister asked her if she was depressed or sick. She was not having much fun on the vacation she needed so badly but felt okay. On her sister's recommendation, she called her doctor when she got home. The next day, after a long morning of tests, she learned that she had diabetes. She was shocked. She knew something was wrong but never imagined that she was that sick. She knew nothing about diabetes and was terrified. Dorothy had lost her job six months before. She was sure her diabetes was a result of the stress. She had already asked friends and family for support. Now what was she going to do? She couldn't imagine how she was going to afford all the supplies that she needed. She asked, "Why me" and "Why now?" Developing diabetes at a time when so much else was going on and money was tight made accepting it more*

*of a challenge. Dorothy felt burdened and still feels*
*angry about the demands that having diabetes places*
*on her. "At one time, I stopped taking my medication.*
*I convinced myself that I didn't really need the pills,*
*but really I just hated spending the money on them."*

It took her 11 years, most of them spent in denial, but she can say that now she is facing her diabetes, things are much better. She thought she had freedom when she was eating what she wanted to and not thinking about diabetes at all, but it wasn't freedom. In reality she was locked in by her anger and was too tired to do the things she enjoyed. She had to convince herself that giving up eating fried foods every day wasn't going to deprive her of her freedom. She had to realize that taking care of herself was a good thing. "I still feel angry at times, but mostly I get mad at myself for not doing what I need to do."

It is important to connect with your own diagnosis story. It is always an emotional event in a woman's life. When you are diagnosed with diabetes, you are very vulnerable to the suggestions and attitudes of those around you. You may have felt powerful negative emotions at the reactions and attitudes of the health care professionals and your family and friends. You need to recognize how you felt then because these emotions may still color your viewpoint and responses now.

To move through the levels of acceptance, you need to know what level you are on, what issues you don't accept, and what new challenges diabetes may bring you. From here you will be able to develop a more concrete plan moving you toward wellness.

## *Womanhood*

All your life you grow and change with each new developmental phase and milestone. You gain perspective and life experience through meeting those challenges. What you learn in each stage enables you to grow into the next stage. You may need to retrace your steps occasionally to find new ways to move through old issues.

Look through the list of stages that women grow through as they mature. Following the list is an exercise that will help you

# Life Stages

## Getting out on your own
- developing confidence in peers, co-workers, superiors, and community
- conforming to friends
- developing an intimate committed partnership
- deciding about marriage
- selecting and preparing for an occupation
- starting a new job
- feeling lonely
- experiencing pregnancy and childbirth
- leaving home
- experimenting with family values
- achieving independence from parents (emotional, & financial)

## Discovering who you are
- searching for identity
- developing/nurturing partnership
- considering/starting a family
- dreaming about your future
- taking on major responsibilities
- developing satisfying social groups
- working toward personal goals
- deepening friendships
- asking "who am I?"
- doing what you "should"
- making commitments
- beginning/nurturing a career

## Raising questions
- having/raising children
- settling down
- advancing in your career
- accommodating to multiple-roles
- asking "what do I want to do with my life?"
- desiring freedom
- declining satisfaction in marriage/ partnership
- divorce
- recognizing personal limitations

## Changing perspectives
- learning to play again
- experiencing peak competency
- emotional turmoil
- accommodating to limits of personal power
- changing careers
- moving
- asking "what about me?"
- changing physical activity
- parenting teenagers
- asking deep questions
- remarriage
- having a sense of aloneness
- awareness of mortality
- death of a person close to you

**Enjoying more freedom**
- experiencing menopause
- beginning to consider/plan for retirement
- acting on new values
- adjusting to empty nest
- selecting a few good friends
- adjusting to grandparenting
- reviewing personal, relationship, and career goals
- supporting aging parents
- enjoying life
- enjoying more financial freedom

**Deepening sense of purpose**
- softening feelings
- adjusting to limitations
- dealing with financial pressures
- quiet joys
- facing death
- death of loved one/close friend

- making new friends
- loss of energy
- retirement
- developing steady commitments to self and others

**Entering the twilight**
- experiencing loneliness
- depending on those who once depended on you
- seeking companionship
- having trouble with memory
- sense of peace and perspective
- freedom from "shoulds"
- losing partner and friends
- preparing for death
- difficulty getting around
- experiencing physical challenges
- enjoying the present moment

—*adapted from* Kicking Your Stress Habits, *Donald Tubesing, 1989.*

appreciate what you have already lived through and the life challenges you are now facing.

Each phase has its own unique qualities and impact. Let's take a moment to identify where you are and which situations you have already experienced. Draw a line at the stage you are in now. Check off the issues you have already dealt with. Circle the ones you are dealing with now. Be sure to look at the issues in the stages preceding and following the one you are in now. Now, list the specific changes (big and small) that you are currently adapting to.

## Adapting to life change

At each stage in your life, you must adapt to changes. Change always challenges us, but each new challenge is an opportunity. Facing challenges (and opportunities) can be stressful. For example, you left your family as a young adult and set up your own household. Leaving home challenged you to set up and keep house, to organize your finances, and to assume full responsibility for your diabetes. Above all else, and no matter what, you can expect change. It's normal and inevitable. Demands on your time will come and go. Responsibilities shift. Self-image evolves. Friendships wane. Energy fluctuates. Bodies grow and change. All of which influence your diabetes control and your ability to achieve your health goals.

As a woman with a chronic illness, you can expect to be challenged financially, physically, and emotionally. Meeting these challenges can seem overwhelming at times. It will help you to remember that being challenged pushes you to draw on your own wit and wisdom to develop new skills and strategies. You have the opportunity to discover that you can do more than you thought.

Doing what you need to do to care for yourself will help you move through life changes. Keeping regular habits while working on one or two key changes at a time makes the process less confusing. Regular eating, exercise, and blood glucose monitoring habits can do a lot to give you a feeling of control, while you adapt to other changes in your life.

The life skills that you learn in order to cope with diabetes are transferable! For example, bearing the constant financial burdens of diabetes may have forced you to budget more carefully, create a rainy-day bank account, and check your insurance claims, to be sure they were being properly handled. When you retire, these habits will serve you well as you navigate the maze of Medicare and enjoy the money you put away. This is just one example of the training that makes every woman with diabetes better equipped to deal with the expected challenges of growing older. Loretta discovered that growing older has many blessings as well as losses.

*Recently, my very close friend passed away. That has left me sad and scared. I was faced with the reality that I will die, too. For a while I began to question why I should bother with all this diabetes stuff. But then my granddaughter asked me to help her deal with a crisis. I felt honored to know that I was needed and that I could help. I then realized that I had a lot to live for. I know that I will die someday, but I don't have to rush it. There is a lot of living yet to do.*

*The nice thing about getting older is that I don't get caught up worrying about what other people think. I don't need to be perfect. In fact, I have learned to laugh at myself. I really do funny things sometimes!*

Facing life and death is a part of getting older. These challenges are magnified by having diabetes. You can live in fear of this and let life pass you by, or you can accept it and engage in life right now, every moment. Loretta's wiser self allows her to enjoy her quirks. Taking life less seriously through laughter and a good sense of humor is an important tool to balance your perspective on life. Loretta has let go of the need for society's approval. She is comfortable being who she is.

As human beings, as women, and as individuals with diabetes, we move through stages of life and come to new levels of understanding. Your age, stage in life, responsibilities, coping style, and resources play a big part in how you respond to change and how you accept and incorporate diabetes into your life.

## Wellness

Wellness is wholeness—a blend of body, mind, and spirit. Wellness is about consistently making choices that enhance, rather than jeopardize, your health and well-being. It is now commonly accepted that if you approach life positively and do things regularly to promote your well-being, you can affect how well and even how long you live.

As we said in chapter 1, you can have serious physical health problems and still feel well. You are not simply focused on what's wrong with you and getting relief, but on what's right and living to the fullest! Wellness is not simply the absence of illness or injury. It's an attitude and a way of approaching your life. Your personal wellness depends on being tuned in to yourself and seeking care and knowledge in order to thrive. Your regular routines, what you think, and how you react to things are the guideposts along this path. You will need to examine how you react to stress (adversity) and how your reactions influence your physical and mental well-being. Do you take a hot bath at the end of an exhausting day, feeling proud of all you accomplished as you relax tense muscles and foster a good night's sleep? Or, feeling depleted, do you drink a few glasses of wine to unwind, fostering hypoglycemia at 2 A.M. and causing a sleepless night?

## Making Healthful Changes

Living is about change. Each change, no matter how small, opens up new opportunities and challenges. These opportunities

---

### Making Healthful Changes

**Realize**—What belief or behavior do I want to change to enhance my health and well-being?

**Vitalize**—Determine something you can *do* to make this change.

**Prioritize**—Decide how you want to make it happen. Find the necessary time, approval, money, space, or motivation you need. Figure out how you will deal with any barriers that may get in your way.

**Synthesize**—Practice it, refine it, and make it part of you. Incorporate the new belief or behavior into your regular routine and *self-concept.*

**Revitalize**—As this belief or practice becomes out-of-date with your realities, begin the cycle again.

---

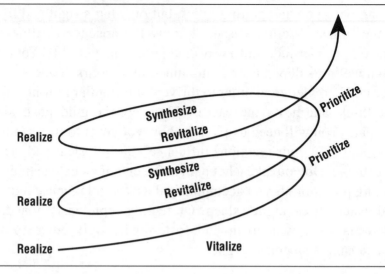

## Diagram of Healthful Change

Prioritize

Synthesize
Revitalize

Realize

Prioritize

Synthesize
Revitalize

Realize

Realize — Vitalize

---

## Self-care Exercise

What was the most recent belief or behavior you changed in caring for yourself as a person with diabetes (for example, starting an exercise program)?

_____

_____

### 1. Realize
How did you become aware that you wanted/needed to do this? Where did you get help in learning various ways to do it?

_____

_____

### 2. Vitalize
How did you decide what to do? Did you list many different ways?

_____

_____

Which one did you choose?

_____

_____

## 3. Prioritize
List anything that you felt would make it difficult to adopt the new behavior or belief. How did you deal with these barriers?

_____

_____

What did you have to overcome or make happen to adopt the new behavior or belief?

_____

_____

## 4. Synthesize
Describe the process of fitting this new practice into your lifestyle and dealing with the barriers you listed above.

_____

_____

What did you learn about yourself in this process?

_____

_____

## 5. Revitalize
What changes have you needed to make to this belief or behavior over time?

_____

_____

_____

test you to discover resources within yourself and your support network, and use them to enrich your life. The process of change is one of realizing what you want and changing your priorities to incorporate the change that will add vitality to your life.

Can you see any life changes in the future that might require you to revitalize your current practice?

Eleanor has type 2 diabetes, diagnosed at age 53. She is now 62, single, and a legal secretary for a law firm. She has had a long-standing relationship with a man five years younger than she. Two years before she was diagnosed, she was told that her blood sugar was a little high. She started a walking program that helped her bring her blood sugar down by the next time she went to see the doctor. She thought that she was okay.

> *I was happy with my work and all that I managed to accomplish in my life. But I had reached a point that I wanted someone to take care of me. I was tired of doing it all alone. I wanted someone else to decide what to eat. Or to shop or cook without me having to ask. I would have loved for someone else to make decisions. I have no children to rely on. My parents were elderly at the time and not able to help me. Then I was diagnosed with diabetes. What a blow! It was one more thing that I needed to take care of.*

Eleanor was responsible for managing her home, paying the bills, doing the cleaning and cooking as well as planning the social calendar. She was pleased about her career but she realized that she wanted to do more for herself. Diabetes added to her sense of urgency, demanding more attention and expenditure of energy. Being diagnosed was vitalizing to her in paying more attention to herself. It gave her the push she needed.

> *With the diagnosis, I began to watch what I ate. My job was very demanding, calling for extra hours over the weekend, but I managed to bring the computer home and complete my work after taking a lovely long*

*walk. This demand conflicted with my intentions to
exercise and carry out my routine chores. For a while
I watched what I ate and started walking again, but
my job got in the way. Between taking care of my
home, paying attention to my boyfriend, and working,
I didn't take time to exercise. It was kind of easy to let
exercise go because it isn't something I enjoy. Finally,
I asked my supervisor to hire an assistant. Now I am
in control of my workload. I made a rule to never go
into the office on weekends.*

*It is still a mystery to me why I don't do what I need
to do. Even though I know better, I still don't follow
the meal plan or exercise as I could or should.*

Managing diabetes depends on Eleanor changing old habits in eating and exercising. Any attempt to make a change is important.
However, to make lasting change a woman must truly want to do what
is necessary. You have to break through your natural resistance to
change.

It is also important for Eleanor to let her health care provider know
when the treatment program isn't working for her. She may need more
medication or to start on new therapy. The critical thing is not to let
blood sugar stay out of control too long. By paying attention to her
blood sugar levels and monitoring changes in how she feels, she can
keep in touch with her diabetes and her body. Intentions to change
behavior are great, but if unfulfilled, they don't do any good.

We all move through predictable phases when we change. We
resist, we explore, we experiment, and sometimes adopt. We move
in, move through, and move along. Whether the change was
planned, (like deciding to wear an insulin pump), or unexpected
(like being suddenly diagnosed with diabetes) these same phases
occur. The most profound changes usually occur during predictable
life changes such as adolescence, the consummation of a relationship, the birth of a child, and menopause; and during life events
such as the death of a loved one, a move, a job change, any change

in family composition, or a serious health problem. If you are not satisfied with how you cope with or respond to these events, get support and adopt some new coping strategies that work better for you.

Angie was diagnosed with type 1 diabetes when she was 13 years old. She is now 34, the mother of two girls, and works at a local school as a teacher's aid. Currently she is going to school to become a special education teacher with a focus on hearing-impaired students.

Let's look at Angie a year ago. She was on the treadmill of life. She was trying to develop herself intellectually by taking two classes a week, while trying to meet the needs of her husband, children, and house. She would fit diabetes care in wherever she could.

*I was 15 pounds overweight. I had struggled to lose weight after having my children. I took insulin twice a day. However, on busy days I often forgot my shot and took it after breakfast and sometimes, hours after dinner. I checked my blood sugar when I felt funny and treated low blood sugar when it occurred. Otherwise, I didn't have the energy or take the time for self-care.*

She was and still is committed to being a good mother, wife, and companion. The needs of her family and home conflict at times with all her other needs. The "superwoman syndrome" lurked in the background and slowly drained her of vitality. She had forgotten to include herself on her list of priorities.

Maintaining friendships and letting people know about her diabetes was always an issue. She had so little time for friends and feared being judged by her peers.

*I didn't have time to go out with my friends. I had forgotten what it was like having a heart-to-heart talk with a friend. I hadn't been out shopping or to the movies in ages. I didn't even have time to go on a date with my husband! I felt guilty because I didn't spend enough time with the kids. I didn't know who I was. I felt isolated and alone.*

Even though she was busy and surrounded by many people, she felt isolated. Angie's health began to suffer, requiring her to stop, reflect, and develop a different approach.

*I had frequent vaginal infections, was tired all the time, and cried at the drop of the hat. I was snapping all the time at my kids. School was more difficult. I knew my life was out of control when I became unconscious because of low blood sugar and required treatment in the emergency room. My marriage was tense. My kids suffered the most. I was cranky when I was high and just plain irritable when I was low. I felt so bad.*

Angie was disconnected from her body and her spirit. Dividing her time into so many pieces diverted her attention from noticing what her body was telling her. She ignored the muscle aches and the messages that she was on overdrive. She just kept pushing and pushing until exhaustion and severe hypoglycemia slapped her in the face.

Today things have changed.

*I am learning how to take some time for me while still caring for my family and teaching. I have had to learn that I can share some of the responsibilities with other people, and I don't have to do everything on my own. I am learning about quality time with my family. Now that they are older, it is a lot easier. Being a good mom doesn't mean being with my kids all of the time. I worked with a diabetes team who started me on three shots of insulin. Surprisingly enough, it is easier because I am less likely to have low blood sugar during the middle of the night. I now check my blood sugar 2–4 times a day for four days out of the week. I talk to the nurse every two weeks. She helps me adjust my dose. My kids even help remind me to take insulin. I even let them stick my finger. I never thought about getting my kids involved. The diabetes educator helped me figure out how to include them. I think it's a good thing.*

*I also see a dietitian who is helping me to lose some weight. I really haven't liked my body. I just didn't have the energy to plan healthier meals. Eating on the run was our life!*

Angie's self-care program included much more than taking insulin and checking blood sugar. She negotiated with her husband to share some of the daily routines to give her some time to get out with friends and to exercise.

*I now start the day by waking earlier to do my "diabetes thing." I also mentally think about what I need to do that day. My husband helps to get the kids ready for school two days during the week, so that I can go for a walk with a friend in the morning. Together, he and I have divided the chores in the house. He is giving a lot. I really appreciate it. I have a little more energy to pay attention to us as a couple. We are beginning to have some time together again. We go out on a date about once every two weeks, grocery shopping! I have a friend watch the kids for two hours so that he and I can have time together. I know I need to exercise more but I'll deal with that in the future!*

Sharing the tasks and responsibilities has enabled Angie to conserve her energy and focus it on the most important parts of her life. Sharing has allowed her to protect her most valuable asset, herself. She is beginning to honor herself and to respect her needs.

Angie realized that she had to reorganize and refocus to feel well. With support, she was able to identify how she could share self-care responsibilities with her family. She is learning how to use the skills and talents of diabetes care professionals so that she doesn't have to carry the burden of diabetes herself. It isn't always easy, but it is a healthy approach.

## Chapter 4

# Relationships

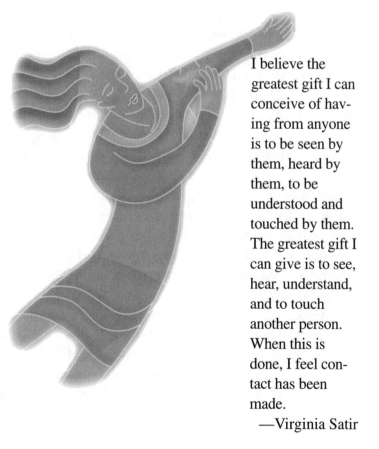

I believe the greatest gift I can conceive of having from anyone is to be seen by them, heard by them, to be understood and touched by them. The greatest gift I can give is to see, hear, understand, and to touch another person. When this is done, I feel contact has been made.

—Virginia Satir

Seeking the best life has to offer and wanting to give your best to the people you love is a great reason to polish your communication and negotiation skills. The desire to be there for the people you love is one of the most powerful incentives for taking care of yourself. As you age, grow, and develop, you will redefine what *being there* means. But it always involves listening and connecting with the people in your life. The truth is that being there for your self is essential to being able to be there for others. Improving your skills in relating to others will also improve your ability to tune in and respond to your own needs.

Communicating effectively is a vital life skill. It supports you in building strong relationships with the people you love and in getting your needs met by the people who are there for you. It will also help you to work with health care professionals to develop a treatment plan that matches your needs, resources, and lifestyle. In this chapter we explore what being supported and being supportive is all about. We examine how you can build more meaningful relationships using communication strategies.

It can be very lonely living with diabetes. Mutually supportive relationships help dissolve this loneliness. Allowing another person to support you opens a door for you to support them in ways they may otherwise never experience. Giving and receiving support builds trust between two people. This trust strengthens the relationship. Your ability to create and nurture relationships will be tested as you move in and out of new situations. When you decide to confide in another person, how he or she perceives diabetes may determine how he or she relates to you. Some people may choose to shy away from you out of fear and ignorance. Worse, you may shy away from them out of fear of rejection or being misunderstood.

Developing meaningful relationships may be the single best way to promote your well-being and prolong your life. Having relationships with people who are supportive is basic to your health. Maintaining these relationships requires confidence, trust, and interpersonal skills. Gaining the skill and confidence necessary to deal with the strains that diabetes places on your existing relationships takes practice. How, then, do you acquire these necessary skills? It is not realistic to expect to get this training in a routine doctor's visit, so you need to take the responsibility for acquiring these skills on your own.

In chapter 1, we looked at how women view having diabetes. You need to look closely at what having diabetes really means to you and how it influences the way you relate to others. Then you want to check the other person's understanding of diabetes and provide them with accurate information. This can clear up a lot. Modern medical and nutritional advances have liberated you to lead a more independent life. People who are not familiar with diabetes don't know about these advances. The average person's perception of life with diabetes comes from a time when being diagnosed with diabetes meant bleak prospects. This is not true today with blood glucose monitoring, a wide variety of medication options, new medical tests to identify complications early, and more ways to treat them. To separate fact from fiction, it is important for you to stay current with diabetes developments and share what you learn with others.

Once you have gained comfort in sharing what you need to say about having diabetes, you will be better able to take on other things that influence your relationships.

## How Does Your Personality Shape Your Relationships?

Each person has a unique personality made up of traits that shape our beliefs, influence our behaviors, and generally color our lives. It does help to be aware of our personality quirks, so we can work with them instead of having them work against us. Here is a list of personality traits that you may want to cultivate to make your life with diabetes flow more smoothly. No one automatically has all these traits, but just being aware of them gives you a standard to aim for in most situations.

## Helpful Personality Traits

**Personality Traits**

- ○ Acceptance: loving yourself with all admirable and less than desirable characteristics
- ○ Discipline: following diabetes plan, getting out for the walk, or following the meal plan even when you're not in the mood
- ○ Forgiveness: allowing yourself to make mistakes, to be less than perfect
- ○ Commitment: honoring promises to yourself, following through with intentions despite other requests for your attention
- ○ Self-reliance: knowing how to help yourself get through the day
- ○ Flexibility: knowing how to go with the flow, to change plans at the last minute, to consider alternative ideas
- ○ Creativity: creating solutions to problems—yours and those of others
- ○ Proficiency: possessing the skills necessary for self-management
- ○ Patience: dealing with the unpredictable events in life, the uncooperative blood sugar, and the other people in your life
- ○ Positive self-esteem: knowing that you are worth it—essential when things get tough
- ○ Ingenuity: problem-solving even when the experts are stumped
- ○ Adaptability: meeting unpredictable and crisis situations with flexibility
- ○ Perseverance: never giving up
- ○ Intuition: trusting your inner voice to know what is right for you
- ○ Confidence: feeling capable and sure of yourself
- ○ A sense of humor: seeing the light side and laughing at your mistakes
- ○ Willingness: being open to new ideas
- ○ Openness: involving family, friends, partners, and health care providers in aspects of your self-care

Knowing and valuing who you are as a woman influences how you view others and communicate with them. This is not to say that having a positive attitude ensures there will be no problems. But it does improve your ability to handle the problems as they arise without compromising yourself or your sense of integrity. The more you consider yourself in a positive light, the more apt you will be to seek out assistance when you need it, listen to your own good sense, follow through on taking the actions you choose, and enjoy a feeling of well-being.

## Your Support Network

People range in the type and quality of support they can offer. Each of us has unique ways of acknowledging and accepting real support. The same is true for rejecting or ignoring other support that we find unacceptable. In any successful interaction, information is communicated, emotions are expressed, and an understanding is reached. It is your responsibility to get your point across, to handle your emotions, and to make agreements that work for you. Which people in your life support you? Who interferes? How easily do you relate to them?

In the box on the next page, list the people or groups of people in your life now. Include partners, children, relatives, friends, work and volunteer associates, and other people who are important to you.

Go back to your list. Circle those who generally support you and underline those who don't.

What are your reactions to your list? List those emotions in the space below. Acknowledge these and think about how you would like to feel about each person on your list.

_____

_____

_____

_____

_____

## List of the Support People in Your Life

Intimate partner _____

Children _____

Friends _____

Family _____

Work and/or volunteer associates _____

Health care providers _____

Others _____

Your feelings about people who are there for you and about those who are not can color your own view of having diabetes and affect how you handle it. You cannot change another person. But you can change yourself. Expand your own interpersonal skills and try out new ways of relating to others. There isn't one right way to support another person or accept support from them. Each person that you listed above has a unique relationship with you, understanding of what you need, and style of helping you.

> *Susan still vividly remembers a stranger she counts among the most supportive people she has ever known. Just released from the hospital, hungry and exhausted from her recent surgery, she attempted to maneuver the cafeteria line with her luggage. As her blood sugar dropped rapidly, she was overwhelmed by the task of buying lunch. The attendant saw her need, called another attendant to cover the register, picked up Susan's tray, and escorted her to a nearby table. She*

*placed Susan's tray on the table, put her luggage on
a nearby chair, and said, "Have a good lunch."*

Someone really cared and helped Susan in a time of need. Almost nothing was said between the two women, but the warm compassion expressed by a stranger will always remind Susan that people do care. Support comes in different ways. Look at all the many ways that you are supported.

Now think of the people you turn to for the types of support listed on the next page. Write their names next to the roles they play in your life.

How do you define being supportive? How do "they" define being supportive? Everyone reacts differently to another person's attempts to listen, understand, and help them. What feels supportive for one person can be irritating for another. Letting others know what is supportive to you makes it easier and more rewarding for them to help. Sometimes this is difficult and will strain even the strongest relationships. This is when clear communication and fair negotiation can make a big difference in your relationship and comfort.

Diane feels frustrated by the financial burden of diabetes. Jerry is worried, not about money, but about the impact of Diane's diabetes on her. Actually, this problem is aggravating the existing communication problems in her relationship.

> *The cost of diabetes supplies, medical bills, and exercise classes is a burden. Our finances are drained by diabetes. I want to be a normal mom and to provide for my children. Sometimes I feel guilty diverting money away from doing something for them to do something for me.*
>
> *I don't want to be a burden to my husband, Jerry. He does so much.*
>
> *Jerry admitted being afraid of her diabetes, wanting to help but feeling helpless. "I don't know what to do*

*for her. If I could, I would take it away. I don't dare to ask her how she feels or tell her that I am concerned about her choices in eating because she will think that I am a nag. I wish I knew what to do."*

Sacrifices must always be made. This is not easy work. Communicating honestly with a loved one can also be very difficult. It takes courage to admit that you can't do it all alone. It also takes courage for your partner to admit his concerns without hurting you. Frank discussion between you and your partner depends on you. Take the risk and give someone you care about the chance to tell you how much they care. From time to time, you may need the help of a family counselor to help you over the rough spots.

## Dealing with Other People

Living with diabetes, you will be faced with dealing with other people, their perceptions about you, your diabetes, and the choices you make in managing your health. Other people's ideas of what is right for you may or may not make sense to you.

Samantha is struggling with other people's comments.

*People have so many misconceptions about my actions and my diabetes! Whatever I put in my mouth seems to be monitored by other people. I can't tell you how many times I hear "Are you supposed to eat that? Be careful, you might get complications." How am I supposed to feel after that?*

*You know, sometimes I tell people that I am low as an excuse to eat something "sinful!" Otherwise I have to deal with a barrage of opinions, arguments, or questions. At those times I get defensive. I already feel guilty. They just reinforce what I already know. It is like putting salt in the wound. It isn't as if I don't want*

## Who Do You Turn To?

For cheerleading _____

For help with personal problems _____

For direction and clarification _____

For expert diabetes advice _____

To share problems _____

For respect and approval _____

For energy and motivation _____

To provide for you (financial, housing, food, etc.)

_____

_____

For inspiration _____

For an honest opinion _____

Do you feel supported by the people you listed above?

_____

_____

Who do you shut out when he or she tries to help?

_____

Who offers support in a way that you really appreciate?

_____

_____

*to do what is right; I just don't do everything perfectly all the time. It makes me feel like a little girl again!*

*I was brought up to be a good girl. To be a good girl and have diabetes means to have good HbA$_{1c}$ levels; not to cheat on my diet; and to follow the rules! There are times that I don't do what I should, and I feel guilty. Sometimes I like to forget that I have diabetes.*

It is natural for people to comment on what is going on in our lives. Sometimes these comments are motivated out of concern, sometimes they are not, but they leave us needing to set boundaries about what we will accept. It is natural to reject people's efforts to help when they are not useful, or are even irritating to you. Again, clear communication helps others know what you really need from them, even if it is just letting you vent or share space. It is your responsibility to tell other people what you need. It is especially important to tell them when they really have supported you. This strengthens your relationship and gives them the joy of feeling that they were there for you.

If you look at it from their point of view, you may realize that trying to help you, especially if you are ambivalent about doing what you need to do, is tricky. It isn't easy to offer support that is rejected. It can be frustrating and irritating for them. It is painful to watch someone you love struggle doing something that seems harmful to him or fairly simple to you.

*Roberta dreaded the day she saw coming when her pills would need to be replaced by insulin shots. She swore to herself and her husband, Harry, that she would never give herself a shot. Her anger and stubbornness bothered Harry. How could this woman who raised four children and balanced the finances for his business for 35 years refuse to do what the doctor said? He joked with her about it, but his jokes made her even angrier.*

*Harry thought this task was easy. He didn't realize that the idea of giving herself shots was very intimidating to his wife. This simple technical skill was associated with fear and painful memories for her. Roberta needed to share these memories with Harry. As a small child, she watched her Aunt Harriet give herself shots in the kitchen before meals. Diabetes took Harriet's life, after it took one leg and made her almost blind. After Roberta explained this to Harry, he understood the reasons that she wasn't ready to face giving her own injections. She didn't want to end up like Harriet. Then Harry could be compassionate and help her put things in perspective. Going on insulin will probably help her get better control of her blood sugars, and better control can stop or slow down those scary complications.*

Often women with diabetes refuse to ask for help. Fearing rejection or being put down is common. Needing to appear to be in control often gets in the way of asking for the assistance you need. Having your feelings misread is common. You may not be aware of how you are expressing yourself. Your emotional reactions can be hard even for you to understand. Give yourself time to adjust to a change and turn to other people for help; this is a sign of inner strength.

Getting and giving support in a loving relationship demands clarity in communication. Being loved by another person doesn't mean he or she can read your mind. It isn't fair to expect anyone else to know what you need.

It is also very important to keep in mind that the first step to good communication is being clear about what you think yourself. This can be difficult when you are in the thick of accepting change, or otherwise distracted from clear thinking. Being consumed by strong emotions, for example when you learn you have developed a serious complication can make it difficult to hear what is being said to you or to articulate your concerns. Change is messy and uncomfortable. Talking it out with those who know you well, can help you gain clarity. Another person's more objective perspective may help you gain valuable insight.

Strengthened by other people's nurturing and respect, you can adapt more easily and securely to change. Your part in assisting them to support you is as important as their part. Realize what you are asking of the people who want to support you. Here are some examples of support commonly desired by women with diabetes. Each is followed by a phrase illustrating how the need could be communicated.

- **Be understanding and patient.** "It's not easy to balance all my responsibilities. I would love for you to be more patient with me."
- **Be accepting of me.** "Sometimes I just need time to absorb it all. Hold me and love me for being me."
- **Be positive and upbeat.** "Help me keep my sense of humor."
- **Applaud what I am doing.** "Remind me that I am working hard, even if my glucose meter reads 200!"
- **Be supportive.** "I need to know you believe in me especially when I am feeling overwhelmed."
- **Be involved.** "Let me explain what I am doing to . . . (eat less fat, walk more, keep our expenses down)."
- **Just be there for me.** "I know that I am the one who has diabetes, but knowing you are there makes a real difference. It sometimes helps me knowing that you are willing to be by my side even during the painful times."

## Social Skills for Health and Wellness

Checking your blood sugar is concrete. You do it, and it is done. Relating to people when you are experiencing blood sugar or emotional highs and lows is the real work. Preparing healthy meals is easy compared to relating to a child or spouse who refuses to eat them. The people you relate to—your social network—and the way you relate to them define your social life. Those people who are there for you, no matter what, are as valuable as your glucose meter. Clear communication and negotiation are vital skills for good relations with other people. This work has three parts: clarify what you want to communicate, get the message across, and make agreements to get what you or they need.

## Clarify what you want to communicate

Communication is a two-way street. The better you are at being clear, the easier it will be to get your message across. Take the time to straighten out your thoughts, think about how you want your message to be heard, and reflect on the best time to communicate before you utter a word. This will boost your success at getting your message across. There are a few other elements to consider.

**Deciding whether or not to share information.** Not sharing information is a valid choice. You have the right to choose what you will share and when. But, relationships are based on two people sharing experiences, thoughts, ideas, and dreams. Sharing things that you have difficulty thinking about takes courage. A woman who chooses not to tell a close friend that she has diabetes might be considered rude when she declines a piece of surprise birthday cake. Her choice not to tell makes her responsible for the strain on the relationship. A good way to determine what you need to share and when is to ask yourself, "Does her/his knowing that I have diabetes matter to me or our relationship?"

**Being truthful.** It is hard to admit that you haven't followed your meal plan, medication schedule, or exercise recommendations to the people who care about you. Guilt goes hand in hand with denial and dishonesty. It is so easy to say it like you wish it were instead of how it is. Practicing honesty in your relationships takes courage.

*For 20 years Maria answered her mother's predictable question, "How's your diabetes?" with "It's fine." One day she decided to tell her mother that diabetes and*

*the foot problems it caused were not at all "fine." She*
*explained how painful her feet were, and for the first*
*time, her mother knew how she could help. A friend*
*had raved about how helpful a podiatrist had been,*
*so she suggested that Maria call the podiatrist and that*
*she would be happy to go with her. Maria had never*
*considered seeing a foot doctor and was touched by*
*her mother's caring.*

Friends and loved ones need honest communication from you to help you cope with difficulties. Building a relationship of mutual respect depends on being honest. Working from accurate information will allow your doctor to really help. Health care professionals base their health care decisions on what you tell them. Honesty is a crucial aspect of empowering them to do their jobs. Practicing this may feel awkward at first, but it will encourage your doctor to be honest and give the best care for your health needs.

**Respecting limitations.** Everyone is limited by how much they understand and how well they can respond. It is unfair to expect anyone, including yourself, to do or know it all. Sometimes stopping to think about where another person is coming from and what he or she knows may relieve you from feeling misunderstood and angry. The simple act of asking that person to repeat and elaborate on his or her perceptions will give you the opportunity to learn whether he or she sees things the way you do. At times you will not be able to persuade another person to share your view. Respect this. Work at his or her level of understanding or acceptance until he or she is ready to learn more. This prevents frustration and wasted time.

**Using feedback.** You have the right and responsibility to ask for clarification and assistance in fitting recommendations into your life. Remember no one can know what your life is like except you. You do not have to accept what a health care provider or family member advises, but you do have to decide what is best for you. Keep in mind that the advice or feedback may not be what you want to hear, but it still may be what you need. Your challenge is to understand what is being asked of you, listen to your inner wisdom, and decide how to respond. Anger can arise when we know that the messenger is right, and we don't want to admit it. If you notice anger in your response—it may be a clue that the message is consistent with something that you already know.

Diabetes can affect the way you relate to others and how others relate to you. Marilyn described her life with diabetes as occasionally being surrounded by a well-intentioned chorus of people telling her what to do and how to do it, or criticizing her for the choices she makes. Sofie reports that her daughters often scold her when her glucose targets have eluded her. Comments like these are well intentioned, yet they can feel judgmental and hurtful to you. Have you ever found yourself in a similar situation? Have you felt yourself cringe or flare in anger when you heard similar remarks? If so, you are not alone. The situation and the feelings of the people on both sides are normal. What better time to remember that people need your help to learn how to approach you!

Here are some hints for dealing with others' comments and observations.

- Be honest with yourself about what you are doing and decide whether or not you are acting in your best interest and what to do about it.
- Remember that you are the one making the choices, even when others don't agree. You also have the right not to share all the reasons why you do what you do.
- Be careful not to take what is said personally. Tell this part of your ego to be quiet.
- Take in the suggestions and comments, think about what has been said, keep the ones you find valuable, and discard the rest.
- Consider thanking the choir and telling them that you are happy they want to support you. Teach them how and when to support you.
- Take a deep breath and check in with yourself about how you feel or think about the situation before you react one way or another.

- Remember that perfection is an illusion. You are perfectly imperfect!

## *The language of treatment and words of healing*

How do you view your situation and how do you speak on your own behalf? The words that you and others use to describe your diabetes will affect how you feel about yourself and how others treat you. You may not be able to control the words others choose, but you can control what you do in response to them. One choice is to ignore them; another is to ask to be spoken to more respectfully. For example, after a brief visit with your physician, you hear her say to her nurse, "this brittle, insulin-dependent diabetic needs help with compliance and tightening her control. Could you arrange an appointment with our diabetes educator to review insulin and exercise regimens?" How would you feel? Some people might feel diminished. What could the doctor have said that would have made you feel supported? How about "This woman is really struggling with her blood sugar control. I wonder why things are so hard to manage and what we can do to help her?" It is amazing how being listened to can change a whole relationship, from one of distrust and anger to one of trust and collaboration.

Does your own choice of words influence how you view yourself and diabetes? Yes. Throughout this book we have deliberately used words that convey an attitude of respect instead of those traditionally used to talk about diabetes. These words convey our respect for you. Your choice of words is powerful. It takes time, but using words that reflect your beliefs and values will set the stage for you to grow in the direction you want to go. Using affirmations is an excellent way to do this (see chapter 7). The words you use convey not only what you are trying to say, but also your worldview and your expectations. The first step in improving your relationship with diabetes may be as simple as changing the words you use to discuss it.

Gloria is a 72-year-old woman who has had type 2 diabetes for 12 years. She is married, with 5 children and 13 grandchildren. Originally she was taking diabetes pills. At the time of her diagnosis, she had high blood pressure and high blood fat levels.

*Getting diabetes was a blow. I now realize that I basically denied it for the first three years. Now that my blood sugar is lower, I feel better. I had no idea how bad I felt! For years, I loved to play bingo every week. This got me out of the house and gave me time with other people. I was busy with my family and work. It was exciting seeing my kids get married! At first I paid attention to the diet, but after a few months I started to cheat. I really love food, especially desserts. It was hard not to eat the way I used to. I never liked exercising, so I didn't walk like I should have. I didn't have the time to exercise, or so I led myself to believe! I didn't feel bad, so I thought I was doing okay.*

Work, planning and cooking meals, doing the laundry, and cleaning house distracted her from paying attention to her diabetes and other risk factors. Take a moment to reflect on the words Gloria used—diet and cheat. As we mentioned before, words influence how we give meaning to things. Diet suggests depriving yourself of foods you like and short-term weight loss. It isn't surprising that she only followed her diet for a short period of time. Meal plans bring guidelines for healthy eating into your everyday life, and you choose which foods to eat. It's a way of living and it's for the long term. The meal plan is yours, the choices are yours, and your favorite foods can be included. The term "meal plan" implies a guideline that helps you make food choices. Gloria's words imply pain and suffering. When she chooses to use words like meal plan and choice, it's liberating.

### The process of relating to others

Here are a few things worth considering about building and nurturing relationships.

**Forming new relationships.** Remember that your best friend used to be a stranger. Break the ice by introducing yourself and asking open-ended questions; this is the hardest part. A friendship may grow. Initially it's probably not necessary to bring up diabetes, but trusting another person with this information tends to strengthen relationships. It is easier to bring it up when you are feeling good, instead of waiting until you have to explain an insulin reaction. Relationships are strained when you withhold information that would help the other person understand you.

Sheila, a parent of a six-year-old, still can't talk to her daughter's new school teacher after running into her in a parking lot when her blood sugar was seriously low.

> *I* *have this sinking feeling in the pit of my stomach when I think how confused she must have been. I didn't recognize her or follow her description of how wonderful Sarah was doing in her new class. I can't bring myself to tell her that I was having hypoglycemia. I am so embarrassed. She must have thought I didn't care.*

**Asserting yourself.** Assertiveness may not come naturally to you. Respecting yourself is at the core of being assertive. Through practice, you will become less awkward. You can memorize assertive responses and practice them in the mirror. Don't fall into making excuses or apologizing. The first step is to know what you want from another person. The clearer you are in your own head, the easier it is to be assertive.

> *M*y *friend Alice always chose the restaurant we went to after bingo on Fridays. Her favorite was Lou's Diner. This was a real problem because we always had so few low-fat options. One night when we left the noisy bingo hall, I asked if we could go to a different kind of restaurant that had the foods on my meal plan. She said, "Sure." Why did I wait so long?*

**Listening for the meaning behind the message.** It takes time and attentiveness to hear what another person is saying to you. Listening to the words is the first step. Hearing the intended meaning involves much more. The tone of voice, facial expression, body language, and gestures all add meaning. If you are unclear, ask for further explanations, and listen. Don't respond. Don't defend. The final step is to check with yourself to see whether you are able to hear. Is your head too full of your own issues to listen objectively? You must be able to separate your own emotions and biases from another's. If you find it difficult to do, you might ask for more clarification, ask more questions. Get more information instead of getting emotional. Your emotional and physical state will affect what you hear. Being aware of this contributes to clearer communication.

**Ways to get your message across.** Say it over the phone. Announce it at a dinner date. Let him know on a long walk. Write it in the sand. Call her at home when you both agree on a good time. Sing it. Write it. Fax it. E-mail it. There are many ways to convey a message. Choose a method that you are comfortable with and that suits the other person. This makes success more likely.

## Negotiating for What You Need

Negotiation is what people do each time they make an agreement. From deciding what's for dinner to working out your diabetes treatment plan, people are making agreements. The way you handle the interaction that leads to the agreement is negotiation. Many things influence this, but there are some definite people skills—making eye contact, staying in the room until an agreement has been reached, or clarifying what you will compromise and what you will not—that can help you arrive at agreements that meet your needs.

### Dealing with conflict

Deborah Jones, a trainer in negotiation and problem-solving skills, points out three common mistakes that can derail negotiations.

**Being scared off or turned off by the other person's approach to the problem.** You never get to the problem itself. Common ways of approaching a problem are: avoiding, accommodating, competing, compromising, or collaborating. Each has good and bad points. People tend to favor one or two of these under pressure, and there is almost always pressure coming from somewhere. Be aware of each other's styles. If you dislike the other person's style, it can derail the negotiation.

**Forgetting to ask why we want what we want.** You may know what you want, but do you know why you want it? Does the other person? Do you both have the same interests and goals? Try to avoid getting into a tug of war over options. Try to discuss the reasons why an option is your favorite one.

**Not spending enough time discovering the differences between the two parties.** Conflict is inevitable, and it is always an opportunity to learn something valuable. Be willing to discover and discuss differences. You need this information in order to change and grow. Try being creative instead of spending valuable time arguing over a solution.

## *Basic negotiating skills*

### Working with confusion and emotion
- Think through your goals for the relationship by asking yourself what would be right between you.
- Be "hard" on (angry at) the problem and "soft" on the people involved. Separate the people from the problem.
- Reject insults. Firmly confront a verbal personal attack without leaving the negotiation. For example, "When you _____, I feel _____, which will only make it more difficult for us to succeed here/ solve the problem/address your concern about _____."
- Ask yourself what you imagine (it may or may not be true) about this other person, and then ask what is causing you to imagine it. Say, "I see you _____, and that causes me to imagine _____. Is this true?"

## Defining the needs of both people
- State the problem.
- State what your desire is, even though you are not sure how to achieve it at this point.
- Actively listen. Restate what you believe the person has said—what he wants, his concerns, or his desires. Ask him to repeat to you his understanding of what you have said. Let him know how correct he is.
- Directed listening. State what you want, your concerns, and your desires.
- Clearly come to an agreement about what the problem is before either of you criticize or propose solutions.

## Generating options—ideas to choose from
- Be firm on *interests* while being flexible about options.
- Stop the other person from mixing up the process of generating options with deciding among them.
- Explain that listening is not the same thing as agreeing.
- Encourage a discussion about possible scenarios of each position or idea.
- Agree to disagree and to come back to it later.
- Determine whether you have all the information that you need.

## Considering fairness
- Ask what she would do in your shoes.
- Ask her what she thinks would be fair in this situation. Find out why she feels that way.

## Choosing among the options
- Explain how the solution you like could be a good solution from his point of view, too.
- Explain how the solution he likes could help you.
- After you have brainstormed a list, note the ones that help both of you. Could you live with any of the others as well?
- Make a final agreement specific enough so that both of you know exactly what to do and when.

## *Interacting with professionals*

Developing a trusting relationship with your health care providers is critical to your long-term success. This may work differently for different women. Some women click with the one doctor that they have. There is mutual trust, respect, and good communication between them. Others find that they struggle.

Viewing the professionals in your life as allies instead of gods will be a relief for both of you. You all have meaningful roles, limits, and areas of expertise. Your involvement in this relationship is very different from those with friends and family. You are seeking professional care and paying for it. The more you can do to find professionals you respect, who share your beliefs about health and health care, the easier it will be to communicate with them.

The patient–professional relationship is a two-way street. You have the right to expect guidance, respect, and a partnership. You are the expert on you. You also have the responsibility to follow through with your provider's recommendations and to communicate when it is challenging or not working. Sharing your thoughts and fears is important because they cannot read your mind.

Having a healthy relationship with your doctor and other health care providers calls on you to be an advocate for yourself. At times you may need to disagree with your provider, to question, or to persevere until you are heard and your concern is addressed. It is true that some women do encounter difficulty being heard and understood. If this type of relationship continues, it may lead to feelings of frustration, anger, and distrust. Women deal with this differently. Some doctor-surf (go from doctor to doctor) seeking that one person who will really listen. Others get angry and give up—on the doctor, the treatment program, and even themselves. Please don't let your physical and emotional health suffer! If you find yourself feeling or acting in this way, this is a danger sign. You are at risk. It may be time to seek the help of someone who can be an advocate for you, someone else who can speak on your behalf, address the issue with you, and help you find other alternatives. It may be time to find another health care provider.

Ideally, you will have one primary care physician who takes care of your general health needs and coordinates care with other specialists. This person should take the time to talk with and listen to you, help you plan ahead to prevent problems, prescribe medications carefully, be available by phone, have your trust and respect, and know about all of your health problems. A provider's qualifications and interpersonal skills, the office location, and ease of scheduling appointments are also important for you to consider.

## *Interviewing your doctor and health care team*

If you have the opportunity, we encourage you to interview your health care providers to determine whether they are going to be a good fit for you. Do you feel comfortable with their beliefs, biases, or practice style? Here are some areas you might explore. Think about other issues that are important for you.

- Who's on the health care team? Does your provider have the type of support people, such as nurses or dietitians, that you might need when you have a question or problem?
- Will you be referred to other specialists and do they work well together?
- How does the provider communicate issues to you and your other doctors?
- What are the provider's beliefs and experiences dealing with diabetes complications, menopause, breast cancer, pregnancy, or heart disease?
- What are the provider's beliefs, biases, and experiences dealing with various treatments such as hormone replacement therapy, insulin pumps, or alternative therapies?
- Does the provider like for their patients to ask questions about current therapies or questions about other therapies?
- When you have a concern about something, and it is in between visits, how do you handle it? Who is available to address your concerns and questions if you need immediate assistance?

The type of relationship that you have with your provider is critical to your comfort and health. Remember that you are worth the time it takes to address your concerns, your symptoms, or your questions. You have the right to know the pros and cons of all the options available to you. You have the right to seek different opinions and to be treated with respect. Sometimes personalities don't mix. That is okay. Move on. It may take time to find the right fit. Keep your options open. It is possible that no single provider can meet all your needs.

There are a number of issues—real or imagined—that may influence your relationship with your health care providers. We mention a few here along with suggestions about how to enhance the relationship so that it is more fulfilling for you.

**Understanding what is said.** Some women have difficulty absorbing and retaining information that their health care providers tell them. They only think of questions to ask later, after the visit.

- **Ask your provider to write important advice down.** Take notes so that you won't forget. Hearing and understanding are two different acts. You need to take responsibility for requesting clear explanations from all health care providers. Ask them to tell you again, and write it down. Getting over your pride when you can't follow what your health care provider is saying is the first step. They are not judging you; they are only trying to help.

- **Consider bringing another person along** to help you hear the recommendations, to ask questions that you may not think to ask, and to support you if there is a disagreement. Members of your family or a close friend may want to help you this way. This may be hard to ask for, particularly for us superwomen who think that we should be able to do it all on our own.

- **Go prepared.** Getting ready for a visit with your health care provider involves more than just deciding what to wear and how to get there. You need to be prepared to describe your concerns in ways that she can understand. Take the time beforehand to carefully review your reason for seeking help. List your questions and concerns. Note what you think caused or influenced the problem and other factors influencing it.

This practice builds a relationship based on mutual respect and responsibility.

- **Seek out other professionals.** Consider seeing a nurse educator or dietitian, who can help you understand the information.

**Feeling intimidated.** Many women feel intimidated by the doctor, especially when they feel that the doctor is pushing a particular therapy. Some are reluctant to express doubts, disagree, or even ask questions.

- **Bring someone else** in to the visit, someone who can help you understand why the doctor is considering a particular treatment and help you communicate why it isn't comfortable to you.
- **Ask questions** about the risks, the benefits, and the alternatives. Get information and weigh your options.
- **Gather information from other resources.** Discuss your questions and findings with your doctor or other members of the team. You have the right. It is your body and your future.
- **Get a second opinion.**

**Feeling minimized.** Some women believe that the provider minimizes their experience and just doesn't make time for them.

- **Confront the issue with the physician.** This may feel awkward but does not need to be disrespectful. Be clear about what you need and what you want from the professional caring for you.
- **Consider finding another doctor** who better fits your needs, who listens and answers your questions.
- **Reach out to other members of the team** who might be able to intervene on your behalf or at least support you as you work with a particular physician.

**Helping them understand you.** Some women feel that male physicians cannot relate to their experiences.

- **Respect their opinions.** While male health care providers cannot truly have female experience, that doesn't mean that they cannot understand and be sensitive to your issues and concerns. It is an individual thing. Gender is only one aspect of a provider's capacity to relate to you and serve your medical needs.

- **Look at the situation from their point of view.** Are you helping them help you?
- **Ask for information** to check out your opinion and theirs.
- **Trust your instincts.**

**Getting to choose your provider.** Some health insurance programs limit your options.

- **Ask for your provider services to be covered.** Increasingly, insurance companies are determining who can take care of your medical needs and how. Their interest, like yours, is to keep you healthy. If you like the person who is taking care of you, and your insurance company limits your access to this provider, find out who your representative is and ask whether your doctor can be included on their list of preferred providers.
- **Ask to speak to the medical director or case worker** who is most suitable to hear your case. This may not be possible, but don't give up easily. Persistence often pays off.

The reality is that communication with any health care provider is complex. There are times that you can do it. There are times that you will need the assistance of someone else. There are times that you need someone to restate what you have been saying in a way that the health care provider understands. There are other times that you need someone to interpret and restate what it was that the physician or nurse has said to you! Health care is changing rapidly, so try to get into the spirit of "experimenting" and don't let your feelings get hurt.

**We believe that you deserve a health care provider who**
- allows you to express your fears, concerns, and needs
- listens and hears you
- involves you in the process to the degree that you feel most comfortable
- respects you and your choices without making you feel small or ashamed

- problem-solves with you, tries new things, works with you as a partner
- is able to admit that they do not know and suggest you get a second opinion

*Trudy, a 68-year old woman with type 2 diabetes suggests that the right doctor is the one who knows he doesn't know everything, respects you as a human being, and has a zest for life himself. She says, "He is the one who knows I am a princess!"*

## Making use of resources for getting the support you need

While your health care providers are the first level of support for helping you handle your diabetes well, there are other sources of support for you.

**Classes and support groups.** Simply being with other people who are on the same diabetes pathway is enormously uplifting. You feel understood and you can gather strategies from other people living with diabetes. This provides a kind of support found nowhere else. Find a group by calling local hospitals or the nearest American Diabetes Association (ADA) chapter found in the white pages of your telephone book or check the ADA web page at www.diabetes.org.

**Books and magazines and the World Wide Web.** Reading is one of the best ways to learn something new. There are many sources of information that can help you learn and grow. Look for information that is written and presented in ways you can easily understand. Ask support people for their advice on books that might help you. You may be amazed at how much has been written for people working on the same challenges that you are.

**Agencies and organizations.** There is a rich network of organized groups whose purpose is to offer assistance. Finding an agency to assist you takes some effort on your part. Agencies are more aware of each other than you probably are of them. So, asking one agency representative to suggest who else might offer assistance with a problem is a good idea. The phone book is a good place to start finding out about local and state agencies.

**Health insurance providers.** Insurance companies do a lot more than pay your medical bills. Read the literature they send you. Ask whether they discount or cover services such as health club membership that may help you meet your wellness goals. You should have an insurance representative. It is that person's job to communicate with you about the services the company offers and to resolve any problems you are having.

**Other resources.** What other resources might you want to consider using? Have you considered working with diabetes educators to develop your diabetes skills or attending a local college or community education program to hone those life skills that you want to develop further?

Over time you may find that your skills are not enough to reach your current goals or to meet the new demands in your life. Your body will change, resulting in changes in blood sugar levels, medication needs, and overall blood glucose control. As things evolve, our strategies must also evolve. Diabetes skills may need updating, or you may need a new treatment program. Diabetes providers can help you adjust your medications so you can dine out without experiencing hypoglycemia or help you design a more flexible daily schedule. The experts and teachers in hospitals, colleges, and community centers serve as your external coaches. They can help you brainstorm a new strategy or fine-tune an old one.

## Putting It All Together

A woman needs to communicate in ways that help others understand her needs and desires. She also needs to clarify goals and intentions for herself so that her communication is clear. Critical to her ability to maintain integrity is her ability to listen to others' suggestions, to weed out what works and doesn't work, and to seek out the assistance of others when needed. In seeking out information, a woman needs to analyze and discriminate what to believe from the media, literature, and others; to question and persevere until the information feels right; and to feel secure enough to know when to continue in the search and when enough is enough. Yes, we are suggesting that you be curious about and in charge of your life.

When you treat yourself and the people around you with attention and respect, your relationships will enrich your life. Relationships with all kinds of people who can care, nurture, share, support, guide, mentor, teach and love you are priceless. They will support and sustain you through it all.

# Chapter 5

# Body, Mind, and Spirit

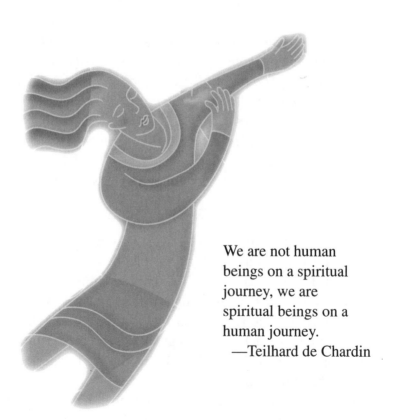

We are not human
beings on a spiritual
journey, we are
spiritual beings on a
human journey.
  —Teilhard de Chardin

L iving with diabetes is not just a matter of numbers and physical events. It affects how you live in your body, use your mind, and experience your spiritual essence. Diabetes becomes another path to self-knowledge and connectedness. This chapter is about using the wisdom of your body, mind, and spirit to support you in enjoying a meaningful life. Every woman is motivated by something that she considers special. Being around to see her grandchildren grow up and get married makes a difference for Loretta.

*I want to see my grandkids get married! So I have to take better care of myself. Now I see a doctor regularly and respond to my needs promptly. I had a small problem with my eye, and I went to see the eye doctor right away. I didn't always do that.*

*When I am motivated or feel good about myself, I tend to exercise more. My husband is my coach. He doesn't let me get out of walking. He tells me that the dishes can wait until after we get back. I spend a lot of time with my children and grandkids. I love to go shopping with my daughter. That is a great diversion from eating.*

*I guess you could say that I keep a positive attitude, and . . . (pause) I try.*

Loretta has faced many physical and emotional challenges. All of these trials and tribulations have helped her to stop and reflect on what is important in her life. This awareness drives her to get out and walk and to stop eating after she has had two cookies. She has also learned to rely on her support people to help her. Being there for her grandchildren has given Loretta the reason to take better care of herself. This is infectious. Seeing her desire motivates her husband to be there for her.

Have you ever wondered just how much having diabetes influences who you are and how you act? Have you ever had a sinking feeling after a spat, thinking that maybe your blood sugar was to blame for your negative remarks? In the same way, women commonly question their emotions in relation to pre-menstrual syndrome (PMS) and menopause. You could say to yourself, "I am easily irritated, so I'll test my blood sugar. This is the way I tend to react when my blood sugar gets above 250." The more you learn to rely on your own internal wisdom to cue you into your body or state of mind, the easier it will be to experience wellness.

It takes practice. Getting to know your body is like getting to know what a newborn needs. First you look at and listen to the baby cry, and then you try to satisfy her with a diaper change, feeding, or rocking. After a lot of trial and error, you begin to notice subtle differences in her cries. With experience you develop a routine, meeting a loud high-pitched cry with a feeding and a quieter cry with a cuddle. In time you will be able to decipher your own body's language, whether it is sweaty palms, dry mouth, muscle tension, headaches, cramps, or low energy, in the same way. Your responsibility is to stop, take a deep breath, and determine what the headache and muscle tension might be telling you before you decide how to react.

Let's take some time to work with this.

As a person with diabetes, you have a unique tool—your blood sugar—giving you insight into your body's messages. Your blood glucose level affects and will be affected by what you think, what you feel, and what you do. Often, you will know about and respond to a need brought to your attention by an elevated blood sugar rather than by any bodily or emotional discomfort. For example,

- your shoulders are tense after working long hours
- after a week of fluctuating blood sugar levels, you are tired when you take care of your grandchildren
- you are thirsty, after having high blood sugar for a few days

Your initial reaction may be to ignore these symptoms. It is bothersome to focus on things you cannot always control. In some instances it is healthy not to let discomfort slow you down. This is discipline. Other messages cannot be ignored (like heart-attack symptoms) because they indicate that you are at immediate risk. Most messages are more subtle. Chronically ignoring these signs and symptoms can lead to serious problems down the road. You need a way to determine which bodily signs to respond to and when. This is a critical skill in diabetes self-management. By learning to understand what your blood sugar numbers mean in terms of signs and symptoms, you begin to gain a sensitivity that makes it easier to manage your diabetes and be well.

## Taking notes

Writing down how your body feels when you know there has been a change—such as increased stress, low or prolonged high blood sugar levels, or during your monthly cycle—will teach you to notice the effect of this change on your body. This is awareness. Being aware of yourself is the basis of self-care, emotional strength, and spiritual connectedness. Only by listening to your body can your mind and spirit thrive.

Regard blood sugars as a barometer. They remind you to stop, listen, and reflect on what's going on inside you.

> *Rachel reflects on experience with her menstrual cycle, "It slows me right down. Cramps are a good reminder that I need to make some adjustments and tune in to the wisdom of my body."*

Fluctuations in blood sugar can be viewed in the same way. High or low blood sugar certainly causes you to slow down. This opportunity for reflection is all too often missed by women. Instead, we tend to focus on guilt, worry, or frustration and hastily move on before we learn from the experience. The next time you experience a pattern of high or low blood sugar, reflect on what your body might be telling you. Ask yourself whether you are pacing yourself. Is this a signal to nurture your body? In what ways can living with diabetes serve you as a woman?

# Consider Your Body

Let's take a moment to look at how phenomenal your body is.

- The combined pulling strength of all the muscles in your body equals 25 tons.
- Your heart pumps the equivalent of 5,000 to 6,000 quarts of blood through you every day.
- Your ears can discriminate among more than 300,000 tones.
- Your brain, many times more complex than the most advanced computers, operates on the amount of electrical power that would light a 10-watt bulb.
- Your eyes can distinguish nearly 8 million differences in colors.
- The surface area of your lungs is 1,000 square feet—20 times greater than the surface area of your skin.
- Your bones manufacture 1 billion new red blood cells every day, replacing old ones at a rate of 1.5 million per second.
- Your circulatory system is more than 70,000 miles long.
- Your digestive tract is 30 feet long.
- One cubic inch of your bone can withstand a two-ton force.

—Lonny J. Brown, PhD, in *Self Actuated Healing*

This complicated structure you live in is a true miracle. Thinking for your pancreas is an amazing task to be given. Treated with respect and honor, your body could provide you with a lifetime of awe. Living each day so that your body organs and systems can operate at full potential sure makes more sense (and is more fun) than just following guidelines to get the right numbers on your $HbA_{1c}$ lab report.

Your body is the tool you use to relate to the world. You modify it to work for you, and you adjust your life to fit its abilities. The way your body functions will influence how you perceive and respond to all your experiences.

Diabetes can challenge your natural ability to see, feel, and sense the world around you. Knowing your diabetes and your body well enough can help you become aware of any changes. It heightens your ability to pick up internal cues signaling conditions, such as infection, stress, or hormonal changes. Developing this ability to sense what is going on in your body will help you better understand what affects you. When you react to a cue, you will usually choose a reaction that promotes wellness. We seldom think that we can choose how to react. We assume that reactions just happen, when in fact, there is time to choose.

Having diabetes certainly influences what you choose to do with your body, such as running a marathon, traveling overseas, or having children. But so do many other things. Setting limitations on what you do with your body is part of taking care of yourself. Determining where to set these limits is tricky. It involves mediating between your desires, your physical and emotional comfort, and your beliefs about what is possible. So many times we decline opportunities for fun and recreation because we are afraid of what "they" think or because we think we can't do it. For instance, you might decline a request to dance because you don't want everyone looking at the way your body moves on the dance floor.

Women are taught to pay attention to external measures, like ideal weight, rather than to listen to internal messages. The measure of your success too often is reduced to your weight, calorie count, and $HBA_{1c}$. These external measures do give you information about what's going on inside you, but they don't tell the whole story. Becoming aware of the internal cues and experiences of our body can be very exciting, even when the external measures or goals are not. We might begin to feel good inside before we show any change on the scale.

As a woman with diabetes you are even more vulnerable to this, because of the extensive amount of health monitoring, checking, and testing that goes on. Having diabetes increases your awareness of all of the things that can go wrong with your body. Health care providers spend a lot of time tuning into what could be wrong, looking for signs and symptoms of the health problems associated with diabetes. So, it is easy to tune out, as others describe your body in terms of a test result, which makes it more difficult for you to tune into the healthy natural processes of your body.

*As a girl of 13, Allyson sat at camp listening to a respected diabetes doctor explain that girls with diabetes should not plan on having babies due to the complications and potential birth defects. All her dreams of being like her mom were shattered. Years later, she decided to get pregnant anyway. Allyson read everything she could get her hands on about diabetes and pregnancy. She accepted her doctor's explanation that her delivery would have to be induced and could easily require a Cesarean section (C-section). She took birthing classes but paid little attention to the details of natural labor and delivery. Just as the blood glucose machine had helped her succeed with the pregnancy, the machine measuring her contractions and her baby's heartbeat told her how her labor was progressing. After 24 hours of induced, nonproductive labor, Allyson was thrilled for the doctor to perform a C-section and bring her healthy baby girl into the world. However, later she felt as though her experience of one of life's most vital moments was reduced to watching a machine and feeling like a statue from the waist down.*

*Three years later at a birthing center, Allyson had a different experience. She was coached to deliver naturally. She came to the induced delivery of her second child informed, involved, and confident that she could depend on her support team. Allyson was aware of the power of her body. She ignored the machines, paid attention to herself, and enjoyed the natural delivery of a healthy baby girl. Even if she had needed another C-section, Allyson was so much more involved with this birth that she knew she could handle it either way.*

*Allyson's first birth experience was shadowed by her fears from childhood. Those fears were calmed by watching the machines, but she was not as involved as she wanted to be with the birth of her daughter. She was thrilled to have a healthy baby but wanted a different experience the next time. With the second birth, she participated more fully in the experience. She heard the messages her contractions communicated and responded with confidence, using the breathing and relaxation skills she had learned. When the time came, she worked in harmony with her contractions to push Rachel into the world. She was completely in this experience.*

*Pat had been on diets since she was 20 years old. After being told that she needed to lose weight, she fell into the cycle of yo-yo dieting. She went shopping for the latest low-fat, low-sugar junk foods and starved for a week, only to lose and regain the same eight pounds. Pat thought of her body only in terms of how much it weighed. She felt good when she lost weight, felt horrible when she gained, and didn't notice much else about her physical self. Pat avoided mirrors and didn't like looking at herself at all. She hated feeling so self-conscious and found herself staying at home more and more. Each weigh-in during her regular visits to her doctor seemed like judgment day. She always had a good reason for gaining the weight after losing it but still felt like a failure. Then, at the age of 56, Pat began to change. She gave up her desire to look like Marilyn Monroe. She cared less what she looked like and more about what she could do. She wanted to spend more time with friends and to travel. A group of friends from church convinced her to join their informal swimming group. Reluctantly, she went and enjoyed being with friends, so she kept going. She decided to join the local recreation department with a friend, and after six months of swimming, she found that she felt better. Swimming felt good. She began to notice that she spent less time fighting her body and more time enjoying her friends.*

If you strive to measure up to external standards, you always have to look outside yourself to see whether you have succeeded. This doesn't honor you and usually sets you up for failure. When you trust yourself, and listen to your own wisdom, you can define and enjoy your own successes. You are your own authority. This is how to live a more connected and fulfilling life.

If you've never tried to exert yourself much, or are sure you have lost it physically, your self-imposed limitation can become rigid. You may be beyond even thinking of going for a swim or to a dance. Convincing yourself that you are unable to participate in things that are fun for you takes the spark out of life and the spunk out of you. How you think about your body is the basis of how you determine your own limits. And, generally, you can do more than you think you can! Get up and dance!

---

### Your Body

The abilities of my body that I can depend on include...

_____

I am fortunate to live in a body that...

_____

I am limited by my body because...

_____

If I could change one thing about my body it would be...

_____

---

Consider the answers given by Irene, 58, an avid gardener who worked in a local greenhouse. The abilities she could depend on include

> . . . *being able to lift almost anything and rarely getting even the slightest cold.*

She felt fortunate to live in a body that

> . . . *had great stamina allowing her to work long hours in her garden. She loved the time she spent there and enjoyed the reward of seeing things grow.*

She felt limited by her body because

> . . . *her vision was affected by retinopathy, making it difficult to see at night. She hated not being able to go out to bingo the way she used to.*

She would like to change

> . . . *her hips. They have always been much bigger than she wanted. That had always been a difficult thing for Irene.*

What do you think about Irene? Can you see your body as clearly as you see hers? Are you gentle and accepting in your view? Can you begin to see how realistic your own views are and how achievable your expectations?

## Body Image

Having a healthy relationship with and respect for your body is critical for every woman, especially the woman with diabetes. Developing this relationship is very challenging in our culture where the images of women are not based on healthy reality. Our society is obsessed with thinness. This obsession has lead to the presence of two extremes: anorexia and obesity. Women are never satisfied with their body, feeling that they are either too fat, with hips too big, breasts too small, eyes too narrow, or wrinkles too many.

Women are always comparing themselves to fashion models who weigh 25% less than the average woman. The media image of the "ideal woman" is impossible for most women. This leads some women to extreme attempts at weight control, such as starving or poisoning their bodies. Many women feel so frustrated that they discard any effort to keep their bodies healthy, and they overeat. Some women engage in anorexic or bulimic behaviors, exercise to an extreme, or manipulate medications to promote weight loss.

For women with diabetes, this dance is more complicated and potentially life threatening. It is not surprising, because managing diabetes requires so much attention to food. Women are always hearing recommendations to limit fats, to distribute calories more evenly, to avoid eating too much, or to lose weight. Under the constant scrutiny, eating can become an unpleasant experience. And the body becomes the reminder that things are just not right. Frequently unresolved issues about food or weight surface, complicating a woman's commitment to maintaining diabetes control and following the treatment program.

Some women find it very easy to gain weight when they have diabetes. Insulin is a hormone that helps the body to build fat tissue as well as to hold on to the nutrients the body needs. If a woman is not well informed about how best to balance food with medication and exercise, she can easily gain more weight than is desirable. If a woman with diabetes tries to lose weight without guidance, she can easily begin having many low blood sugars. This can lead to a cycle of recurring lows, requiring more calories that eventually result in more weight gain or a weight plateau. This can be terribly frustrating.

For some women, having to limit the amounts or types of food leaves them wanting more. It's common to feel guilty when "cheating" on a diet. The word cheat sets many women up for frustration, guilt, and shame. In response, some women choose to overindulge and abandon their self-care efforts. Others choose to restrict calories, depriving their body of needed nutrients. Black and white thinking results—women feel that they are either on or off their meal plans, good or bad. Good and bad get defined in increasingly rigid terms that would be hard for anyone to maintain long term.

The majority of women with diabetes, who struggle with eating and weight, struggle with a subtler form of disordered eating than anorexia and bulimia. These are the women and adolescent girls who reduce or skip their insulin doses in order to rapidly lose weight. They have learned that by intentionally running their blood sugars high, they can lose weight because most of their calories are lost through sugar in their urine. This is an extremely dangerous practice. Women who do this are at very high risk for diabetic ketoacidosis (a potentially fatal condition). They are also at much greater risk for developing depression, both from the chronically high blood sugars and from the secrecy and shame involved with maintaining this behavior. Research has shown that continuously skipping or reducing insulin over long periods of time places people at much higher risk for diabetes-related medical complications like kidney disease, eye disease, and painful neuropathy. Help is available within your diabetes care providers or with mental health practitioners who specialize in the treatment of eating disorders.

Any preoccupation with your body weight and size that interrupts how frequently and what type of nutrients you put into your body or your commitment to follow your diabetes treatment plan is a call for help. Whether or not you label your relationship with food as having an eating disorder doesn't matter. Any time that food becomes a source of pain or shame, a woman needs support and guidance from professionals who are trained to help them face the issues that cause this struggle. It is complex and no one can do it alone. No matter what method or reason a woman might use, experts understand that hidden pain and unhealed wounds lead to unhealthy relationships with food. If you find yourself facing this battle, we hope that you reach out for the professional support that you deserve. A solid, supportive health care team, including a mental health professional and dietitian, can help you gradually set more realistic, attainable goals and safer ways to cope with your eating and weight concerns.

Learn to honor your amazing body and protect yourself from believing the unhealthy media messages, which idealize unhealthy and unnatural body shapes.

Bulimia is characterized by recurrent binge-eating (the rapid, uncontrolled consumption of large amounts of food). Purging may occur with self-induced vomiting, laxatives, diuretics, insulin omission or reduction, fasting, severe diets, or vigorous exercise. People with bulimia maintain near normal weight and appear to be healthy, yet they often realize something is wrong. Bulimic behavior usually begins in adolescence or early adult life and strikes women in much greater numbers than men.

### Signs of Bulimia

- exaggerated concern with body shape and weight
- a sense of secrecy and shame
- abuse of purgatives
- depression
- changes in appearance
- weight changes
- abnormal interest in food
- severe dieting and exercise
- substance abuse

Anorexia is self-imposed starvation resulting from a fear of fatness. Many women with anorexia are preoccupied and dissatisfied with their body size and some specific feature of their physical appearance. They constantly believe that they (or parts of their body) are fat even though they are obviously underweight or even emaciated. Anorexic behavior usually begins during adolescence. This disorder strikes women in greater numbers than men.

### Signs of Anorexia

- distorted body image
- reduction in eating
- extensive exercising
- social shyness or isolation
- poor self-esteem
- excessive weight loss
- overuse of laxatives/diuretics
- absence of menstruation
- cavities and gum disease
- extreme sensitivity to cold
- hair, nail, and skin problems
- growth of body hair
- denial of problem

Bulimia and anorexia, if left untreated, can lead to many other physical problems and illnesses—even death.

Jenny is challenged by caring for her diabetes while trying to reach an unrealistic body shape and size.

*I never seem satisfied with my weight. Because I am short, I feel I should also be petite. But I am not. I am a size 12, when I want to be a size 6. My diabetes makes it harder. I know that better blood sugar control will mean that it is harder for me to lose weight or even keep my weight where it is. I'm also afraid that if I do not take care of my diabetes, I will feel lousy, my kidneys might fail, or I might go blind. I know that I will feel guilty and that other people are going to blame me if that happens. Sometimes I feel that I cannot win!*

*I get really angry that I have to eat when I don't want to. Like when I have to treat a low blood sugar or prevent one. I resent not being able to eat what I want when I want!*

Diabetes treatment programs do set up a schedule of eating and medication taking. Eating just to prevent low blood sugar can take away from the pleasure of eating and cause weight gain. Jenny is also frustrated that her body shape doesn't match her desire to look the way she wants to. On one hand, she wants to lose weight, and on the other she wants to pay attention to her diabetes control. One seems to make it difficult to do the other. It seems easier not to try. Her dilemma is familiar to many women with and without diabetes. Yet her goal of being a size 6 is unrealistic. Genetically she is not meant to be that size. Striving to do this will always cause her problems.

*I know that if I don't pay attention to my health and ignore it all, I will only feel horrible. I really need a lot of help letting go of my desire to be a size 6. One part of me knows that is unrealistic, yet the other part of me is just dying to be that size. Since I have had this obsession, I have been miserable and basically no fun to be with.*

After careful consideration of the pros and cons, Jenny has decided to focus on her health. She has realized that her physical and emotional well-being are not going to improve if she ignores her diabetes. Jenny now works with a professional to help her redefine her body and weight goals. Now she is focusing her attention on how to be fit, instead of thin. Instead of focusing her attention on feelings of deprivation, she focuses on what she is able to do. She is learning to think of her body more gently and to be more accepting of what she sees. It is taking time but slowly she is learning to give herself more positive messages and to celebrate her body.

## Consider Your Mind

Your mind works in harmony with your body and your spirit to make sense of it all. Through your body you experience the world. Feelings give you clues about what these experiences mean to you and the importance they have in your life. Knowledge can help you interpret your experiences. Your spirit gives you perspective about these experiences in the world beyond what you can see.

The diagnosis of diabetes, onset of complications, an identity crisis, or the death of a loved one are all losses and are followed by the grief process. All of us grieve our losses. This is a normal adjustment to loss and the changes that result. The stages in the grief process have been defined by Elizabeth Kubler-Ross as denial, anger, bargaining, depression, and gradual acceptance. It is common to go back through previous emotional stages when you have to work through new challenges or rework old ones. It is also common to get stuck in a particular stage of grief. If this happens, your energy to take care of yourself or pay attention to your other responsibilities may fall. Seek professional help if you feel you are in trouble.

You also experience a wide variety of emotions related to living with diabetes every day. These range from elation to despair and are as unique as you are. Check off the emotions you commonly feel in relation to having diabetes.

| | | | |
|---|---|---|---|
| ○ shock | ○ sadness | ○ fear | ○ curiosity |
| ○ anger | ○ pride | ○ boredom | ○ nothing |
| ○ depression | ○ frustration | ○ anxiety | ○ happiness |
| ○ deprivation | ○ satisfaction | ○ resentment | ○ relief |
| ○ gratitude | ○ guilt | ○ regret | ○ balance |
| ○ satisfaction | ○ happiness | ○ embarrassment | ○ joy |

In the box below is an exercise to help you examine your emotions about diabetes and the effect they have on your behavior. There are two steps to this exercise. Step one is to list the emotions you feel about the listed aspects of diabetes. Step two is to think about how each emotion causes you to react and write it down. For example, Audry feels angry after getting herself out to exercise and having serious low blood sugar each time. Her emotional response to exercise is anger. Her reaction is not to exercise.

List the emotions you feel in relation to the words listed below.

| Emotions and Behavior | | |
| --- | --- | --- |
| Word | Emotion | Resulting Impact On Your Behavior |
| A cure | _____ | _____ |
| Pancreas | _____ | _____ |
| Me | _____ | _____ |
| Meal plan | _____ | _____ |
| Blood sugar testing | _____ | _____ |
| Family support | _____ | _____ |
| Future complications | _____ | _____ |
| Current complications | _____ | _____ |
| Injections | _____ | _____ |
| Exercise | _____ | _____ |
| Pregnancy | _____ | _____ |
| Health insurance | _____ | _____ |

Is there an overriding theme to the emotions you have listed? How do they influence what you think about yourself, what you feel, and what you do in response? What can you do to gain mastery over your emotions and not allow them to control how you react or behave? They can have a huge impact on the way you feel, take care of yourself, and interact with others.

## You Are What You Think

| Positive self-image | Negative self-image |
|---|---|
| Acknowledge diabetes exists. "I am worth it." "I must take care of myself." | Denial of disease. Shame, guilt, blame. |
| ↓ | ↓ |
| Choose to adopt some healthy behaviors. | Unhealthy behaviors. |
| ↓ | ↓ |
| Handle the ups and downs. Move through the periods of sadness and discouragement. | Negative thoughts about self or diabetes. Sabotage self-care efforts. |
| ↓ | ↓ |
| Seek training to become more aware of choices and support during a difficult life challenge. "My needs and desires are important." | Complain: "Why me? I can't do all this." Unhappy. Waste energy on feeling like a victim. Dead-end behavior. |
| ↓ | ↓ |
| Negotiate treatment strategies with the health care team. "I am uncomfortable with this meal plan. It doesn't work for me. I need something else." | Isolation, pain, loneliness. "They just don't understand." Decreased energy for self-care. |
| ↓ | ↓ |
| Encouragement: Feeling good about the small accomplishments. | Discouraged: "It will never get better." |
| ↓ | ↓ |
| Emotional and physical needs being met. | Progressive physical or emotional health problems. |
| ↓ | ↓ |
| Positive feelings about self. | Denial, shame, guilt. Negative feelings about self. |

# Consider Your Spirit

*We stake our lives on our purposeful programs and
projects, our serious jobs and endeavors. But doesn't
the really important part of our lives unfold after
hours—singing and dancing, music and painting,
prayer and lovemaking, or just fooling around.*
—Father William McNamara

Your spirit encompasses all that gives your life real meaning.
Seeking meaning and purpose in life is an important part of being
human. Finding meaning and purpose to your life gives you peace
of mind and the motivation to be fully involved in your life. In her
book *Living with Diabetic Complications*, Judy Curtis reminds us
that having peace of mind rather than bodily health as our primary
goal allows us to focus on what really matters.

Dreams of the future can provide motivation for taking care of
yourself. Maggie, who is 39, can see herself as a healthy 68 year
old, going to school, and learning new things. She loves children
and hopes to help young people reach their potential.

*I keep trying. When things don't go right and my blood
sugar is all over the place, or my health is bad, I might
cry or grumble a bit, but then I deal with it. I have
found a wonderful doctor and a diabetes educator
who work with me. I also learn as much as I can. I'm
no longer fooled by thinking that knowledge is enough.
Knowledge doesn't take care of this disease. My
actions do. I have to change my behaviors if my health
is going to be the best it can be.*

*I am no perfect being though! Sometimes I give myself
permission to just let go. Not for long, but I decide
when I am going to eat differently or to skip exercise.
It gives me the break that I need. Also, when things
are really crazy, I look at ways of simplifying my life,*

*at least for a few days or weeks. This helps me reconnect with myself.*

Being aware of your vision for the future helps you keep on track. It can give you the motivation you need to keep going. Maggie has also made a valuable connection with a health care provider who works well with her. She feels heard and listened to. She's right that just knowing what is needed to be well isn't enough. Applying what you know and changing behaviors or attitudes into healthy, positive ones is the key.

---

### What Really Matters to You?

List the things you most like to do or the activities that have the most meaning to you.

_____

_____

Complete the following sentences by writing down the first thing that comes to mind after reading them.

1. Life would hardly be worth living if it weren't for...

_____

2. If I could change one thing about my life at this point, it would be...

_____

3. I keep myself alive and energized by...

_____

4. What I like best about myself is...

_____

---

5. I feel most powerful when...

_____

6. I feel discouraged about life when...

_____

7. The one thing I want to do with my life is...

_____

8. To do this, I need to take care of...

_____

Now look over this list and think about what brings meaning to your life. This is the foundation of who you are. It has evolved from your life experiences, values, and interactions with other people. And it will always be evolving.

Motivated by the desire to participate in her grandchildren's lives and afraid of dying early, Gladys is trying to make up for lost time. She was always so worried about what dire event would happen in the future that she didn't live in the present.

*As a young child, before blood glucose monitoring was available, I didn't expect to be able to reach my life dreams. I was afraid that future complications would interfere with the length and quality of my life. I felt the need to accomplish everything yesterday because I didn't think I would be able to do what I wanted in life. I focused on what might happen, but in despair, I haven't taken care of myself. Now with a clear vision of what I want to happen, I am motivated to take care of myself. Seeing my children grow up is important to me. I want to be there for them and for their children. I want to celebrate the good times and share the tough times. I won't be any good if I keep up this pace.*

Gladys is on the treadmill of fear, caught up in the "what ifs." She fails to enjoy the present and misses out on the small miracles that happen around her every day. Her concern has been fed by people around her and statistics that say people with diabetes die earlier than people without diabetes. These statistics were true in the past. With better tools for managing diabetes available, it is now possible for women with diabetes to live long and fulfilling lives— if they pay attention to their needs today.

Gladys lost sight of what was most important to her, her children and her husband. Fear compromised her diabetes control, her relationship with herself, and the relationships with her husband and children.

If your life has meaning, you work with it instead of trying to run away from it. When you are in touch with what really matters, you are motivated to do the work that is necessary to achieve and maintain wellness. For example, getting the best care during pregnancy is motivated by the desire to ensure the health of the baby and by the value you put on nurturing human life. Regular exercise and attention to blood sugar management is motivated by wanting to feel well and the value you put on good health. Or you may be motivated to make better food choices, not by weight control, but by a desire to see your grandchildren grow up and the value you put on participating in your family.

Finding meaning is probably the most personal and difficult challenge anyone can address because there are no rules for how to do it really, except that it requires looking within and searching your soul, which is frightening for most people. It is not something that another person can do for you. However, there are some things to keep in mind.

1. Learn to look within first and trust what you find there.
2. Focus on what is right now instead of what was or what might be.
3. Work toward greater honesty and clarity in your relationships with other people; be just who you are, not who you think you are supposed to be.
4. Work through the pain of loss, instead of allowing it to control you.

We do need to learn to listen to our inner voice. This voice is influenced by the messages that you give yourself and also by the messages that others give you. Meditation, exercise, prayer, and worship are some of the ways that women choose to quiet themselves to connect with and strengthen this voice. Positive affirmations or positive self-talk are important ways to feed your mind and body and harmonize with your soul. Listening to your inner wisdom gives you a foundation for making decisions, dreaming, and planning for the future.

Stop and think where you want to be in 5, 10, or 25 years. Ask yourself, "Am I doing what it takes to get there?" and "Am I giving myself positive messages to support my commitment and intentions of being well?"

You can change the perception that diabetes is a disaster or that it limits you, if that's how you see it. Everyone has challenges of one kind or another. And from the soul's point of view, you might entertain the perception that a challenge like diabetes is a good thing, a great way, perhaps, to learn how strong and flexible and capable you are. You can be whole spiritually, emotionally, physically, and socially. Coping with the daily challenges of diabetes can teach you how.

Ask yourself, "What else can I do right now to feel better about who I am?"

Ask yourself, "What could I do in the future to help me accept this part of me and build a more positive self-image?" Your dreams for the future have a better chance of coming true when you have a vision of where you want to be and a sense of the abilities and talents you can depend on to get you there.

## Harmonizing Your Body, Mind, and Emotions

The body, mind, and emotions are closely connected. More than the body is affected when your blood sugar goes haywire. Frustration easily rears its head. Many hidden factors influence glucose control, too. Getting angry or uptight can raise blood sugar levels. This may be a time to change your treatment strategy, soak in a hot bath, or go to the movies with a friend. Above all, don't forget to keep your sense of humor and to be kind and gentle with yourself.

Diabetes challenges women physically and emotionally, as Bea has realized.

> *P*hysically, I am challenged when I have high or low blood sugar. My energy is sapped, and I don't feel like doing anything. Low blood sugar interferes with my thinking ability and leaves me feeling incompetent. Actually, I can't follow discussions and lose my train of thought. My emotions depend on my physical functioning. When I try to do what I need to do for myself and it doesn't work, I get discouraged. The lack of success with the physical stuff influences my emotions. I try to think that I am in control. Then things don't work out and I am left discouraged, thinking what am I to do?

Emotions affect how people feel about themselves and how much energy they have to take care of themselves. Bea found that when she felt good about herself, she was more likely to participate in self-care. When she was down, she didn't.

> *W*hen I feel good about myself, I have enough energy to do what I need to do. I feel like I am being good to myself. That's nice. I don't even resent eating well! When I am feeling down, I have no energy. My blood sugar goes up because I don't feel like eating right or exercising. My mood gets worse. I feel even less motivated to care for myself and even more tired. Depending on how I feel, I sometimes respond to the high blood sugar, sometimes I don't. I get very frustrated because my blood sugar bounces. It is a vicious cycle! I can't always get the sleep I need

*because I need to get up and take insulin. I need to spend some time problem-solving how to fit my diabetes treatment schedule into doing what I want to do. For example, sleeping in late conflicts with taking my medication on time.*

Self-care takes energy, patience, and time. In the best of times when a woman feels good and has energy, she can manage the crises or scheduling challenges. She does have the capability. However, it is more difficult when she's fatigued, bogged down by high blood sugar and feelings of helplessness. This is a good time to problem-solve other options with health care professionals or friends who can help her discover some new options to try. Think of it as a friend helping you out of the fog that gathers on a path that you travel every day. We all need a little help sometimes.

You may have noticed that women of the 21st century are beginning to create their own circles of women who can support them as they integrate the wisdom of their body, mind, and spirit. Our ancestors lived in communities where women were strong but relied on each other for assistance with daily living, child rearing, and making life transitions smoothly. Perhaps wiser than we, these communities, or circles, created rituals that allowed women to express the wide array of emotions and experiences in their lives. They allowed women to honor the woman within. Joan Borensenko refers to the center of the circle as the heart and the inner light. It is the place where a woman can hear the guidance from her wiser self. Circles, whether you find them in support groups or therapy groups or just groups of friends, are places where women can share their stories. Storytelling—sharing our dreams and hopes, wounds, fears, and triumphs—provides a vehicle for healing and growing. Our sense of family is about circles. Sometimes we need to create another kind of family, our circle of kindred spirits who can support us in our quest for health, for growth and fulfillment.

*Our deepest fear is not that we are inadequate. Our deepest fear is that we are powerful beyond measure.*

*It is our light, not our darkness, that most frightens us. We ask ourselves, Who am I to be brilliant, gorgeous, talented, fabulous? Actually, who are you not to be? You are a child of God. Your playing small doesn't serve the world. There's nothing enlightened about shrinking so that other people won't feel insecure around you. We are all meant to shine, as children do. We are born to make manifest the glory of God that is within us. It's not just in some of us; it's in everyone. And as we let our own light shine, we unconsciously give other people permission to do the same. As we are liberated from our own fear, our presence automatically liberates others.*

—Marianne Williamson
*A Return to Love*

## Chapter 6

# Embracing Our Physical Health

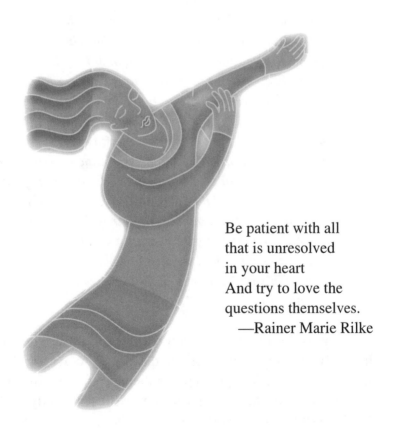

Be patient with all
that is unresolved
in your heart
And try to love the
questions themselves.
  —Rainer Marie Rilke

Whether we are young or old, with and without diabetes, we encounter challenges to our health as we grow older, menstruate, experience pregnancy, menopause, or illness. It is during these times that our body calls us to pay attention, listen, and respond to its needs. We have the choice to get involved with our health, and actively participate in prevention, healing, or treating the problem. Or we can choose to ignore or deny the problem.

*Olivia is a 41-year-old woman with diabetes. She recalls the day she realized that she needed to connect with and pay attention to her body!*

*"One afternoon, the light bulb went off in my head. I realized this is the only body I have. And it isn't a perfect one. I have bulges in places I don't want. I am out of shape and have such low energy. Wishing it were different hasn't made a difference. Imagine that! You know, I have diabetes and a major family history of heart disease. For the longest time, I have ignored the need to exercise. I have been lazy about paying attention to my body—as if it wasn't going to catch up to me! Now I want to make my body strong and be as fit as I can be, so it is in better shape to deal with unexpected events in the future. I figure that if my body is healthier, I might be able to reduce my risk for any problems that could occur. If they do occur, I may handle it better if my body is stronger. I have started exercising with small weights and walking as often as I can. This is the only body I have. I want it to carry me as far as it can."*

Olivia is not unique. It is not uncommon for a woman to take her body and her health for granted. Or to be so overwhelmed with health issues that she just ignores them. To make a difference for your health, you need to get in tune with your body, to become familiar with what nurtures, heals, or harms it. With this knowledge you can take care of yourself. In some ways, you are called to become *full of yourself*—knowing, feeling, listening, and honoring what your body is asking or needing.

This is particularly true for women with diabetes. Having diabetes puts you at risk for experiencing health problems earlier than women who do not have diabetes. Diabetes may also affect how well your body responds to physical challenges such as heart disease, pregnancy, or growing older. If your body is not as healthy and strong as possible, it may not fare as well during the tough times. If blood sugar levels are consistently out of control, that may make it even more difficult for you.

You may see body changes reflected in your blood sugar control. Changes in hormone levels resulting from your menstrual cycle, pregnancy, and menopause may cause fluctuations in blood sugars. This is also true as the body responds to the presence of illness. Diabetes, or blood sugar levels, can be your barometer of how well you are.

In this chapter we explore how diabetes and your total physical health are intertwined. We discuss issues that are common to all women and those that are unique to women with diabetes. We provide you with some insight about the health risks and ways to prevent or deal with the challenges you might encounter. Part of your success depends on whether you include yourself at the top of your list of priorities. Taking care of your physical health, including your diabetes, takes time and commitment and requires tender loving care. Remember, you are worth it!

## Dealing with the Demons

It would be nice if taking care of our physical health were as simple as just doing what is best for us. But we encounter obstacles that interfere with our commitment or willingness to do what we need to do. These obstacles are sometimes internal—our attitudes, fears, feelings of self-worth, and self-confidence. Sometimes they are external—other responsibilities competing for our time, attitudes and beliefs from people we spend time with, and the realities of our challenging health care system. Let's refer to these obstacles as "demons." Success in our quest for health requires that we become aware of the demons as well as develop a healthy attitude for dealing with them. The demons discussed in the next few paragraphs can influence your enthusiasm and commitment. Some may be familiar. You may think of others that we have not mentioned.

## Our sense of worth

To care for our physical health, we need to believe that we are worth the effort. We are worth taking time out of a busy day to prepare a healthy meal or to exercise. Taking time out for ourselves often means saying no to something or someone else. We need to believe that we are important, and it is okay to do what we need to do, even if it means disappointing someone else.

## Self-confidence

Our confidence in ourselves, and in our ability to change when we need to, will be challenged from time to time. When faced with adopting a new behavior, learning a new skill, or changing a long-held belief, it isn't uncommon to find yourself wondering whether you can really do it. Your "inner critic" may try to sabotage your efforts. Take care to speak positively to yourself inside your head and out loud, too. Getting support from people who can reinforce your commitment and coach you may also be helpful in maintaining and building your confidence.

## Expectations

What we *expect* to happen can make us really disappointed or really happy with what actually happens. Periodically, we find that what we can do or what happens does not meet our expectations or the expectations of others. For example, we may have unrealistic expectations about how much weight we can lose in 6 weeks or how far we should be able to walk after a heart attack. If we do not pay attention to our expectations, we set ourselves up for failure. We all know the old saying "You have to walk before you run!"

That wisdom applies to our health, our physical ability, our weight, and our blood sugar control. It takes time. We need to be sure that our expectations about what we can accomplish (and how quickly) are realistic.

### Feelings of fear, guilt, and anger

We are likely to confront powerful feelings and emotions as we face the reality of our physical health. It is common to encounter fears and feelings of guilt. We may put off dealing with a health problem if we doubt our ability to cope with it. Many of us may also feel some guilt, believing that we caused the health problem and berate ourselves with "if only" statements. If only I had done this. If only. . . .

Fear of the unknown can be immobilizing. So much energy is lost worrying about complications or about the future that nothing gets done. Sometimes, fear mobilizes people to take charge and, sometimes, even to overdo. We don't want fear to limit our ability to enjoy life and take care of ourselves.

*Chris, a woman with long-standing diabetes, shared her experience of living with diabetes. So much of her early life with diabetes was spent living in fear and resentment. She said that she wasted a lot of energy worrying about complications and convinced herself that she could never live with those complications! This preoccupation sometimes paralyzed her, limiting her ability to take care of herself and consuming a great deal of energy, which prevented her from enjoying what each day presented to her. Ironically, when she shared her story with us, Chris was living successfully with the complications of renal disease and total blindness. She said that all her worries had done her no good. In fact, she lives her life more fully now, despite these limitations. She has learned about her strengths and weaknesses through facing diabetes and the complications. This knowledge has calmed her and shown her the way to enjoy her life.*

Take-home message

- You are worth the time it takes.
- Take the time to do what you need to do for yourself.
- Living in fear wastes precious energy. Life will pass you by. And if, just if, that which you feared most does happen, you will find a way to deal with it and still be whole.

Somewhere along your path of living with diabetes, you are likely to ask the question, Why? Why me . . . why this complication . . . why did my body betray me? Why? Sometimes there are no answers. Anger is a normal and expected feeling. Anger can be the fuel to move us into action, to take the steps we need to gain control and be involved as much as possible with our care. Anger, however, can also destroy. If you let it burn unchecked or don't deal with it, anger can interfere with your energy, your willingness to believe in your treatment program, and your commitment to yourself. Prolonged anger towards ourselves, our health care team, or the system doesn't do any good. If anger is threatening the quality of your life or your health, you deserve to seek the assistance of professionals to help you work through it.

*Geri has had type 2 diabetes for 14 years. She has two grandchildren and is working hard to get her body healthier. She and her diabetes provider agreed that she needed to lose 10 pounds and to take medication for her high blood pressure. As she began her new activity program and meal plan, she encountered her own inner critic who kept telling her that she would never accomplish this task. She found it very hard to walk for more than 5 minutes. "That little voice inside seemed to always win out. I would give up. Even taking the high blood pressure medication was hard. My mother had died from a heart attack. I kept thinking I was next. I was so scared. Things got better after I finally talked to my dietitian who put me in touch with other women who were dealing with the same issue."*

When you are faced with your own demons, it may be beneficial to share them with others—other women who have encountered similar issues or professionals who can help you deal with the difficult ones. Remember that we are all confronted by demons. It is particularly important to be gentle with yourself as you face your own.

## *Gender bias and gender differences*

Some people ask, "Why can't a woman be like a man or be treated like a man?" This issue surfaces for many women when they deal with the medical community. It is a complex issue. Sometimes, women *are* treated differently from men. Studies have shown that women with heart disease receive fewer procedures than do men. The time between diagnosis and treatment may be longer for women. There are multiple reasons for this. Researchers are learning that women's symptoms of health problems do not always match the symptoms or disease progression that the provider has been trained to expect. A woman is not like a man. For example, a woman's symptoms of a heart attack may not be typical. She does not have the usual symptoms that would make the physician say, "Oh, this is a heart attack."

Until the Nurse's Health Study, which started in the 1980s, most research studied men. This means that the lists of symptoms and treatment approaches that have been tested apply to men and may not always be right for women. Today, more and more studies are being done to look at the differences between men and women. Researchers are finding that some treatments work better in men than they do in women, and vice versa. For example, studies show that cholesterol-lowering medications are more effective in women than they are in men. Women's bodies are still a mystery, and medical science is just beginning to unravel that mystery.

Women are likely to have their complaints discounted as being the result of PMS, postpartum blues, or depression. The reality is that sometimes the symptoms are related to these wonderful states that women experience, and sometimes they are not. Jumping too quickly to the conclusion that the symptoms are related to hormones or emotions may cause providers to overlook an underlying physical ailment. Also, women may encounter this response more often because women tend to be more emotional when they communicate. The health care provider may not be prepared to handle this or have the time to allow the woman to express her whole story. Men are listened to differently because they tend to be less emotional and more matter-of-fact in their communications. This leaves a woman with the challenge to be well prepared for her visit and to learn to communicate her needs clearly and briefly.

Take-home message

- You can communicate your needs and be understood by your health care provider.
- Do not give up trying. Figure out what you want to say and say it.
- Believe in yourself enough to seek help from an advocate who can communicate on your behalf.

## Guidelines for Caring for Your Physical Being

Taking care of our health requires a gentle, realistic, and firm approach. It is work. But we feel that it is worth it. We all have choices. Whatever choices we make, we need to be happy with them. Here are some ideas to keep in mind as you work on enhancing your health and wellness.

1. **It is never too late to start paying attention to yourself.** You can always succeed at achieving a sense of wellness— of being content with who you are. Forgive yourself for the past. You may have made choices that did not serve you well, that increased your risk for health problems. Let that go. There is nothing you can do about it now. Focus on today. What do you want out of life? You may not be able to get rid of your health problems today, but you may be able to pre-

vent them from getting worse. You can feel better. Recall Anna in Chapter 1? Wellness is not defined by the absence of disease. Wellness is a state of honoring who you are just as you are—having a sense of peace and respect, even for the illness part of yourself. Today is a fresh new start. Seek out new ways of reaching your goals in life. Make it count.

> *R*oberta has type 2 diabetes, is on dialysis, and has *heart disease. She acknowledges that in that past she chose to ignore her diabetes and high blood pressure. "I am living today. I have no guilt. I made choices that I cannot do anything about now. If I only have 2 more days, I want to live them well."*

2. **Remember that your physical body may not always cooperate with your wishes and efforts.** It can be very discouraging not to lose weight after working hard to follow a meal plan and exercise program. The body is complex. Sometimes what happens is not in your control. Reviewing your goals to ensure that they are realistic is vital. You may also need a change in your treatment program or approach. No matter what, adopting a healthier lifestyle will make you feel better.

3. **Don't give up.** Even though you cannot change your genetic makeup or control what happens, you do not have to give up. You can increase your chances of success by trying new approaches to keeping your body and mind as healthy as possible. Remember, when you feel like giving up, you might be confronting one of your inner demons that is sabotaging your efforts! Don't give up. Reach out for support in facing that demon. We may also want to give up when things do not seem to be happening soon enough. For some of us, it takes more time to reach our goal than it does for others. As we change a behavior or an attitude, we do not change at a constant rate. Sometimes we hit plateaus, periods of time where no change seems to be happening. During this time, we may need to adjust our expectations and be satisfied with maintaining that

level instead of actively changing. This may also mark the time when taking a new approach is necessary. Consider brainstorming new approaches with a friend or members of the health care team. Whatever you do, don't give up.

4. **Learn to listen to what your body is telling you.** For example, if your blood glucose fluctuates, your weight changes, or your skin begins to dry out, stop and reflect on what your body needs. These symptoms may be telling you that you need to rest more, take time out for a refreshing walk, or drink more fluids. You may also hear your inner voice suggest that the symptoms you have might mean a serious health problem. Work with your health care provider to distinguish real from imagined problems. Your inner voice is your guide. Pay attention to it. This is how you become the expert on you.

This whole book is about making choices and how to get better at identifying and taking care of your needs. We have choices. We can choose to ignore or to respond to our body's messages. We can ignore messages that our body is unhealthy or in pain. We can try to lose ourselves by getting into addictions—eating, drinking, drugging the pain away, or anything that diverts our attention. Recall the discussion in chapter 1 about how ignoring or denying your reality can lead to disharmony and "dis"ease?

On the other hand, you can choose to listen to the body's messages and do something about the problem. For instance, you may finally go to the ophthalmologist to see how serious your visual problems are or to the psychologist to face the painful memories that limit your feelings of self-worth. When you face things that are difficult or painful, you discover your own strength. This is the way your soul grows. This helps you become stronger and healthier.

5. **Learn how to communicate your needs and experiences clearly and briefly.** Practice with a friend stating what you feel your problems are and asking for what you think you need to make you feel better. The other person may not always

agree with your requests. Do not take disagreement as a sign that your presentation or request is not understood or important. Be prepared to discuss your position and be open to hearing the message from the other person. Feedback also helps us make informed choices.

6. **Believe in your own healing abilities.** For thousands of years, people have believed that women are natural healers. Our ancestors were shamans, midwives, and healers of the sick. Reach for the inner healer within you and get to know her. Learn to trust the wisdom and messages from your own body and reclaim your power. Actively participate in your own health. Your inner voice and intuition is your guide! Persevere when you feel something is not right. Learn to put your needs near or at the top of your list of priorities. Being at the bottom of the list will not serve you well!

7. **Own your own risk factors.** Learn as much as you can about your health and your potential for health problems. Choose what you can do to reduce your chances of health problems like heart disease, osteoporosis, kidney disease, and the like. There are some risk factors that you can change. There are others that you cannot. The more risk factors you have for a problem the more likely you are to have that problem. Having diabetes is a major risk for many health problems, especially heart disease. The good news is that it doesn't mean that you are going to have problems. It just means that you have to pay closer attention to those things that you can change. Be aware of your health assets and your limitations as you begin to prioritize how you will spend your precious time and energy.

8. **Seek a health care provider or team of providers who can work in partnership with you,** who consider it their responsibility to help strengthen your innate healing ability. Such a partnership means the health care provider is the advisor who evaluates your health and health risks, informs you of treatment options, and explores with you how you want to apply the treatment options. You are the expert on you. You must

communicate your needs, concerns, and symptoms as they surface and commit yourself to following the health plan you and your health care provider design.

*Vivian has had type 1 diabetes for 28 years. Her attitude towards the many doctors that she works with is to appreciate the give and take. "My doctors are not gods. They do the best they can do with the information that I give them. When they don't hear me, I tell them, 'You are not hearing me!' They are not better than me, they just have a different set of skills and knowledge. I have to respect that. Just as they have to respect me."*

Consider setting up an annual appointment with your providers to explore and confirm what is happening with all parts of you. Make your contacts with your health care provider count. Do your research ahead of time. Give your doctor an idea of what you want or need to discuss so that he can prepare for your visit. Your provider may need to do her own research of the problem or treatment you are interested in, so that she is better prepared to address your concerns.

9. **There are no absolutes in health care.** Recommendations change over time as new research provides information and answers. There is no one therapy that makes sense for all women. In fact, there are several options now available to meet a woman's evolving emotional and physical needs. Determining what works best for you requires trial and error, experiments to find out what works and what doesn't. Working in partnership with a team of professionals, family, and friends can help you explore your options as well as evaluate and modify the approach when needed. Including friends and family who spend time with you and who know you is important because they can support your efforts, show you what they observe, and help you remember and retain information.

To decide whether a particular therapy is right for you involves a process of weighing the benefits and the risks to determine what is best for you. It might require having several discussions with your health care provider about your current health and risk for health problems, the risk for side effects from the therapy as well as some research about the benefits of the therapy. Sometimes, there is no easy answer. Together, you and your provider have to figure your personal risk for a particular disease, such as kidney disease, heart disease, or cancer. Then you will explore what your potential is for developing side effects from the particular therapy. For example, what are your chances of developing side effects of high blood pressure medication? These steps will take into consideration your age, family history, and your own health history. Educating yourself about what is known about the benefits and the risks of each therapy is important. You and your doctor will want to examine the results of studies to determine how they apply to you. Finally, the decision of whether to try the therapy is usually based on the "best guess" of you and your health care provider.

## What Research Tells Us

There are many different types of studies done to assess the risk factors, the benefits and the harm of certain therapies, and the causes of disease. Not all studies carry the same scientific weight. In addition there are many ways of presenting the results. Trying to decide what to believe and what not to believe can be very confusing. We hear about studies that contradict each other. One study shows that a particular product is helpful and another study shows that it is harmful. Or experts raise suspicion about the value of the study or of the treatment studied. What are we to believe?!

The scientific community follows a general premise and you can keep it in mind when hearing or reading about new medical findings. Do not just accept the findings from one study. Before the medical community adopts a health practice or treatment approach, they look at the results from many studies. The more the studies show similar results, the more the findings are believed. We like to believe that studies will answer all of our questions about disease, treatments, and risk factors. However, there is no perfect study that answers all of our questions. In fact, findings from most studies usually stimulate more research to answer more questions.

The scientific and medical communities work hard to determine how the findings from studies apply to the patients for whom they are caring. However, their biases and experiences influence their interpretation and belief in the finding of the study. For example, if your doctor believes that climbing to the top of Mount Kilimanjaro is the best treatment for living a full life, (a bias) then he or she is more likely to suggest this as a treatment approach for you (even when there have been few studies to prove it)!

All people have biases and beliefs. That is human nature. So, it is important to explore with our health care providers what those biases are when we are discussing the results of a study. In this section, we provide a description of two major types of studies and give you information about how to interpret the reported results of these studies.

## Types of studies

Some studies are used to gather information about attitudes, beliefs, and health habits. Others report on case studies. These reports are valuable for physicians and patients because they give information, similar to sharing a story. They do not prove anything but provide more information about potential relationships between risk factors, health problems, and treatment approaches. Other studies offer clues about what might be causing a particular problem. There are two major types of studies that are reported in the news or in the media: *observational* studies and *intervention* studies. They are both valuable but are not the same.

**Observational studies.** Observational studies are sometimes referred to as population-based or epidemiological studies. They involve observing different groups of people and gathering information about their lifestyles, medication practices, health risks, and habits to see whether there are any trends between these factors and health problems. Researchers look at the results to see what differences might account for the difference in health problems between the groups. The results tell us about a potential relationship. They don't *prove* the relationship between one thing and another. They provide evidence that *suggests* a possible relationship. For instance, in the Framingham Heart Study, researchers pooled information on thousands of women and men. They found that the people who had high blood pressure were much more likely to have had a heart attack than those who did not have high blood pressure.

There are many biases that affect observational studies. There is the possibility that the results found are related to the characteristics of the population being studied. For example, people who do not have high blood pressure may also exercise more or eat less fat or just have fewer health problems than people who do have high blood pressure. Women who choose hormone replacement therapy may have other characteristics that lower their risk for development of heart disease. In observational studies, it appears that women who choose to use hormone replacement therapy smoke less, are more health conscious, and have fewer chronic complications than do women who do not use hormone replacement therapy.

**Intervention studies.** Intervention studies are more rigorous. They are often referred to as clinical or randomized placebo-controlled studies. Clinical studies directly compare two or more groups to determine whether one factor causes a particular disease or a better outcome than another. Participants are randomly assigned to receive one of the treatments and are monitored over a period of time to see whether the health problem in those that follow the treatment differs from those who do not. The goal of assigning people randomly to one group or the other is to make the two groups as similar to each other as possible before they receive the treatment. Participants have a 50–50 chance of getting one treatment or the other. For example, the Diabetes Control and Complications Trial (DCCT) was an intervention study. In this study, researchers compared two groups—those who had intensive insulin treatment and those who had conventional treatment—to see which group developed more diabetes complications.

## Understanding risks

The results of a study are usually reported as an increase (or decrease) in risk for a particular health problem as a result of taking a certain drug or achieving a certain clinical state, such as lower $HbA_{1c}$. For instance, people who maintained lower $HbA_{1c}$ levels (had good blood glucose control) in the DCCT experienced a lower risk for diabetes complications than people who had higher $HbA_{1c}$ levels. But there are several ways to describe the level of risk. The reports of studies can be misleading unless you understand how to interpret the results. Risk values give you an idea about whether something is beneficial or harmful for the average person.

In many cases, the study results are reported as a *relative risk*. Relative risk compares a group of people with certain risk factors to a group without that risk factor. For example: Women with diabetes (the risk factor) have more heart disease (the problem) than women without diabetes. The presence of the risk factor diabetes increases the chance of the problem heart disease.

Relative risk also refers to the risk of having a positive or negative outcome in one group of people who are taking a particular treatment as compared to people who are not. For instance, women taking hormone replacement therapy are three times more likely to experience a blood clot than women who do not take hormones. This is the same as a relative risk of 3.0 or an increased risk of 300%.

Now, at first this sounds like a big risk. But in order for this to make sense, you have to ask the next question, "How common is that outcome to begin with?" How common is it for women who do not take hormone replacement therapy to experience a blood clot? Or to state it another way, without hormone replacement therapy, what is the risk for the *average women* to experience a blood clot? This type of risk is referred to as the *absolute risk*. The answer to the question is about 1/10 of 1 percent or about 1 in 1,000 women. So, the absolute risk for experiencing a blood clot for women on hormone replacement therapy is more like 3 in 1,000 women. You can see that when you put it this way, the relative risk—although it is still larger—is not quite as problematic as you might have originally thought.

Let's put them together. If the absolute risk for a certain health problem is high, researchers and doctors get very excited, even when a treatment causes a small increase or decrease in the relative risk. If the absolute risk is low, even if a treatment results in a high relative risk, it doesn't attract as much attention. Here is an example. It is estimated that the average white woman's absolute risk for dying from a heart attack is about 30%. This is a high absolute risk. That means that about 30 women out of 100 will die of a heart attack. If hormone replacement therapy decreases the relative risk by 40–50%, then the absolute risk for developing heart disease becomes 15–20 women out of 100. This is exciting!

As we noted above, it is estimated that the average woman's absolute risk for developing a blood clot is very low—less than 1%. The relative risk for developing a blood clot while on hormone replacement therapy is 3 times higher than for women who do not take it. Because the absolute risk is so low to begin with, this increase—even though it is a concern—tends not to be alarming.

Now keep in mind that relative and absolute risks are based on averages. The risks apply to the average woman and, in many instances, to white women. These studies do not take into account every factor nor are they personalized to you. That is why it is important to determine your personal risk. You and your doctor will need to take an inventory of your current health and the presence of other factors that might put you at risk for a health problem or its side effects. Together you will need to consider the following points before deciding what is best for you.

- your personal health history: the presence of other health issues like diabetes that might put you more or less at risk for side effects
- the condition of your health: whether you are fairly healthy or often sick, whether your health problems are under control
- the types of medication that you take: whether there will be a problem mixing one medication with another
- your lifestyle: whether there are things you do that increase your risk for side effects or decrease your potential for the benefits
- your family history: the health trends and experiences in your family that help estimate your risks for certain health problems or side effects

You and your health care team will need to consider all of these issues as you begin to evaluate whether the results from a study apply to you or are meaningful to you.

You can see that interpreting the results of a study and applying it to yourself involve time and effort from both you and your health care provider. You have to weigh the benefits and the risks. After considering your risk profile (what factors put you at risk for a problem), your doctor may choose not to put you on a certain medication because she feels that you have too much of a risk for developing the side effects associated with that medication. Together you may make this decision even when the study results sound so promising. Likewise, if your risk for a particular health problem is very high, your doctor may recommend a certain drug, even when it has many side effects. He may make this decision because the benefits for the drug in your particular case may outweigh the risks.

## Who is in the group being studied?

Please keep in mind that until the last 10 years, there were very few studies, especially randomized clinical trials, involving women. Therefore, most of the recommendations made in health care have been from the results of studies done of men. What scientists and physicians have learned is that, in some cases, women have different symptoms from men, respond differently to medications and other interventions, and have different risk profiles from men.

In the past, most of the studies that did include women included mostly white women who did not have underlying health problems, such as high blood pressure, heart disease, diabetes, and the like. There are many reasons for this. If the effects of a medication are not really known, researchers do not want to put women in the study who might carry a higher risk for side effects. That would cloud the results of the study and make it difficult to interpret. So, it is important when interpreting a study to check who was in the study population. Are they similar to you? How different are they? If they are really different from you, the results might not necessarily apply to you. You and your health care provider might not be able to draw a solid conclusion. Together you may have to make a reasonable guess.

Thankfully there are more and more studies looking directly at issues relating to women. More national funding is available to look at the unique risks and health problems of women. In the past, it was also difficult to attract women to participate in studies. Women have difficulty getting time off from work, arranging for needed childcare, and fitting the program into their already full schedules. Other women are leery of the health care system. This is particular true for minority women. The scientific community is making efforts to reach out to women. Your help and the help of other women close to you is needed. We need to get more answers to questions such as how women with diabetes differ from women who do not have diabetes. What works and doesn't work? How do African American, Caucasian, Asian, and Hispanic women with diabetes differ from each other? It is up to all of us to get involved, so that we can help uncover the answers to questions about the unique needs and issues of women in health care.

### Keeping it in perspective

When studies show a reduction in risk for a health problem because of a certain drug or behavior, it does not mean that just following that treatment will definitely decrease your risk. Just as there are multiple reasons for a health problem, there are multiple ways to reduce the risk of developing health problems. So if you really want to decrease your risk, it is best to adopt as many health practices as is comfortably possible for you.

## Celebrate Your Sexuality

Women are sensual and sexual beings. Diabetes doesn't change that. One of the most important experiences in a woman's life is to express her sexual desires and to give and receive pleasure. Your ability to experience sexuality is influenced by how you perceive your own worth and physical abilities. To be intimate with others you need to be comfortable with yourself, accepting your body with its imperfections and extra bulges; accepting that your body changes as a result of pregnancy, age, or medication; and accepting your body's needs and desires. You may have to ask for what you need. This is not always an easy task. Developing an intimate relationship with yourself in this way may require facing old wounds, shame, or pain. You do not have to be young, soft, pretty, or delicate to be a good lover or to have a fulfilling sex life.

Women also need a partner who is sensitive and caring. Choosing a partner who fits your style and with whom you are mutually supportive is an important ingredient for experiencing sexual intimacy. Whatever your choice, whomever your partner is, you deserve a partner who celebrates you, stands by you when you face your dark side, and shares in the ups and downs of living as a woman and as a woman with diabetes.

Some women define sexuality simply as the ability to bear children. This definition is too limited and does not value the whole woman. It ignores how important it is to feel fulfilled by the intimacy, pleasure, and satisfaction of two people connecting with each other. Sexuality is as important to a woman in her 60s and 70s as it is to a woman in her 30s.

Sexuality is not just intercourse or a romantic evening with candles, wine, and soft silky sheets. For many women, sexuality is about connecting with another person, sharing expressions of affection, trust, and love. It works best when two people are willing to be vulnerable with each other, tender, and appreciative. In that atmosphere, they can tell each other what they want and explore what gives them pleasure in all areas of their lives.

Women with diabetes can have a healthy and sexually fulfilling life. However, many fear rejection or the negative consequences of future complications. All too often we hear women saying that they feel less attractive or appealing because of their diabetes. A woman is naturally concerned about whether her diabetes will have an effect on her ability to enjoy sex and to satisfy her partner. The older woman who has recently developed diabetes might struggle with the fear that she will be rejected by her lifelong partner. Single and younger women may also share this fear. Having low blood sugar on a date or during sexual intercourse can be devastating to the woman who has not discussed the potential for this to happen with her partner.

The reality is that sexual activity involves physical exertion and can result in a low blood sugar level. When anticipating having sex, you may want to consider reducing the appropriate insulin or you can choose to eat something before having sex. For example, Shelly keeps a supply of raisins near her diaphragm. This makes it easy for her to eat some without having the moment of passion interrupted. If low blood sugar does occur, you may find that you are unable to perform as usual and cannot enjoy the experience. For another woman, being low may enhance her feelings of pleasure. It is important not to ignore the symptoms and to treat them as soon as it is reasonable. To be fair to both of you, it is important to discuss with your partner the potential for low blood sugar, the symptoms, and how to treat it. A negative experience during sex can be devastating to both of you. Openly acknowledging the issue may prevent unnecessary pain. Remember, especially in this case, you are not alone with your diabetes.

# Challenges to Sexual Health

## Emotional

Being able to enjoy the wide range of physical and emotional feelings associated with sexual contact is linked to your emotional state and the nature of the relationship with your partner. Lack of trust in your partner or in your own ability can interfere with your enjoyment. Problems with communication between partners can impact sexual activity. These difficulties can be a result of not knowing each other's needs or preferences. Depression, shame, or a poor self-image may interfere with your sexual desire along with feeling unattractive or disliking certain sexual practices. Seeking help from a mental health professional can be very helpful in dealing with these issues and allowing you to enjoy your relationship even more.

## Physical

The function and health of nerve fibers and blood vessels that feed the female genitals—the clitoris, vaginal wall, and vulva—play a role in your ability to experience pleasure. Complaints of pain or decreased lubrication during intercourse or decreased sexual desire are common symptoms of sexual dysfunction in women of all ages. Using lubricants, learning to relax the muscles around the vagina, or trying different positions may help reduce pain during sex. If you have nerve damage, you may lose some sensation around the genital area. This can lessen your sexual arousal and pleasure.

Women who have multiple health problems may be taking medications that interfere with their ability to have fulfilling sexual contact. Some medications can interfere with a woman's libido (desire for sex), affect the circulation of blood, or affect the function of muscles and nerves involved in the sexual response. Other medications cause drying of the vaginal tissue, which leads to painful intercourse. If you are concerned, be sure to ask your doctor about the effects of your medications on your sexual health and what to do about it.

When you do not feel well, it is difficult to be interested in sex. Eve reports having lost her sex drive. She is dealing with the physical and emotional impact of living with diabetes and heart disease.

> *Sometimes it causes tension between me and my husband. I really love him, but it is just so painful. I don't enjoy sex anymore. He just doesn't understand why. I am not sure that I do either.*

## Does diabetes increase my chances of having sexual problems?

Persistent high blood sugars can increase a woman's chance of vaginitis (inflammation of the vagina), yeast infections, and urinary tract infections. These conditions can interfere with enjoyment of sexual activity even when they have no symptoms. If you have problems with unusual discharge from the vagina, itching, or yeast infections, you should consult with your doctor to determine the best treatment for correcting the problem and improving your blood glucose control. High blood sugars can also zap a woman's energy and sense of vitality. Feeling sluggish and tired can interfere with how attractive and receptive you are to engaging in sexual activity. Getting your blood glucose levels nearer normal will help you feel better and help prevent complications such as neuropathy (nerve damage) and retinopathy (eye disease).

Diabetes complications can affect your enjoyment of sex. Neuropathy and poor circulation may affect the body's ability to respond to sexual stimulation. Living with health problems such as heart disease or kidney disease may deplete a woman's energy. She may fear sexual activity might compromise her health. Usually it is safe for a woman with such complications to have sex, but it may require learning new ways and certainly communicating with your partner about what works and what doesn't.

Women who develop diabetes after their sex roles and marital patterns are established may find that diabetes complicates their sex life. It is possible that the intrusion of the disease and its restricted regimen undermine the woman's self-image, cause major readjustments in lifestyle, and produce or aggravate marital tension. Some women with diabetes have reported that the disease has a damaging effect on relationships and produces more family problems. Emotionally, they experience more mood swings and anxiety than before the disease developed and feel more inadequate and less flexible. Realizing that this often happens may help you keep a more balanced perspective on what is going on inside you.

If you find that you are unhappy or concerned about the sexual area of your life, do not feel ashamed or alone. It may not be easy to communicate these concerns to your partner or to your provider. Yet, if you are to honor yourself as a woman you deserve to have your needs, concerns, and fears addressed. It may mean seeking the support of a counselor sensitive to these issues or a physician who can treat some of the underlying causes.

Here are some issues that you might consider important enough to seek help for yourself.

- a decrease in sexual desire or interest
- vaginal dryness or tightness with intercourse
- pain, burning, or discomfort with intercourse
- pain at penetration or with deep thrusting
- soreness and irritation after sexual activity
- more difficulty reaching an orgasm than in the past
- less satisfaction with your sexual relationship now than previously
- problems in your relationship as a result of sexual tensions
- decrease in self-esteem or emotional pain
- depression

## *Sexuality in the aging woman*

It is a myth that women in their 60s and 70s lose interest in sex or are not capable of enjoying it. Studies and surveys continue to show that many older women are interested in sex and sexually active. In fact, the occurrence of sexually transmitted diseases and HIV are a real concern in the aging population, which indicates that sexual activity is alive and well at all ages.

There are normal physical changes that come with age. It may be more difficult to get aroused, the tissues in the vagina and genitals may become dry or weaker. But you can use lubricants and learn to do Kegel exercises to increase vaginal muscle tone (and improve bladder control). To do Kegel exercises, you tighten, hold, and release the muscles around the vagina. These are the same muscles you use to stop the flow of urine in midstream. In fact, that's a good exercise, too.

In a small study of women 60–85 years of age, the women reported that their attitudes toward sex had not changed much. Sexuality was an important part of their life. It just looked a little different. Hugging, caressing, tenderness, and companionship were as important as actual intercourse. For many, even more so.

Sexuality is an important aspect of all our lives. Physical and emotional intimacy is important to the quality of our lives as long as we live. Sometimes, physical and emotional problems can interfere with how satisfied and fulfilled we feel. When this happens, we deserve to have the challenge addressed. It takes courage and commitment to speak up and work out the details.

## *Menstrual cycles*

You may have noticed your blood sugar values are higher around or during your monthly period. Blood sugars are affected by the natural release of hormones that cause your body to be more resistant to its own insulin or to insulin that you inject. Normally, blood sugar remains high for 3–5 days and returns to the level it was before your period, sometimes gradually, sometimes rapidly. Some women notice this change right before their monthly cycle. Others notice it during or right after. Each woman's body is different.

Your blood sugar can also rise as a result of giving in to food cravings before the monthly cycle. During PMS or menstruation, you might have less energy and not want to exercise. If you stop exercising, your blood sugar may rise even higher. Your ability to control food cravings and to continue with your exercise program will help you balance your blood sugar.

It is important to discuss with your health care provider how to adjust your diabetes medication or treatment program during this time to keep blood sugar levels close to the desired target. Many women choose to ignore this temporary rise in blood sugar. This really isn't the best choice because elevations over time increase your chance for developing health problems and leave you feeling poorly as a result.

To determine the effect of your cycle on diabetes control, you can do some research on yourself. Check your blood sugar 2–4 times a day the week before, during, and after your period for 2–3 months. Work with your health care provider to identify your individual blood sugar patterns in response to changes in hormone levels. This is a great time to also note the effect of alcohol and caffeine intake. Keep a log of your blood sugar, emotions, and intake of fat, carbohydrates, alcohol, and caffeine. Record when you feel better and worse. Explore with your doctor how to make changes in your medication schedule. Don't forget the positive effects of physical activity, relaxation techniques, and healthy nutrition!

### Irregular cycles

Women with uncontrolled blood sugar may also have irregular monthly cycles and acne. Persistent high blood sugar may interfere with the release of hormones responsible for your menstrual cycle. Women with polycystic ovary syndrome (PCOS) may have irregular or absent menstrual cycles. PCOS is a condition marked by excessive production of male-type hormones and insulin resistance. Women with this condition may have excessive facial hair and acne and be overweight. PCOS interferes with a woman's ability to ovulate and be fertile. It is estimated that 5% of premenopausal women may have PCOS. Treatment is important to restore normal ovulation and menstruation. Women with diabetes who have PCOS may also find that they need larger doses of insulin because the body is so insulin resistant. Studies are being done to evaluate the effect of insulin-sensitizing medications on improving ovulation and menstrual regularity.

## Contraception

If you have not experienced natural or surgical menopause (total hysterectomy), you will need some form of contraception, no matter how old you are or what type of diabetes you have. Contraception is particularly important for a woman with diabetes in order to prevent unplanned pregnancies. Whether you have type 1 or type 2 diabetes, planning a pregnancy is vitally important to give your baby a healthy start.

Decisions about the best contraceptive methods should be made with your partner and your physician. You need to take into account your overall health, which method offers the best protection with the fewest side effects, and which one you are most likely to use consistently. You can find out more about contraception methods by talking to your health care providers and checking the resources listed later in this chapter. It is important to choose the right method that works for you! You might want to expand your health care team to include a gynecologist or internist who can work with you and your other providers in determining what methods best meet your needs.

Contraception options range from abstinence to the pill. The best method is one that is reliable, that helps prevent an unplanned pregnancy as well as helps prevent an infectious disease. The "pill" refers to a variety of oral contraceptives made from synthetic forms of two hormones involved with regulating the menstrual cycle, estrogen and progesterone. The synthetic form of progesterone is called progestin. A combination estrogen and progestin pill is slightly more effective than progestin alone (99% as compared to 98% success rate). In the past, a woman with diabetes was advised not to take the pill for several reasons. First, taking oral contraceptives could worsen her blood sugar control. In some instances even today with lower dosage pills, a woman may find this to be true. She and her doctor will need to adjust her diabetes treatment program accordingly, or she and her partner will have to agree on other options. Second, the pill may put her at risk for heart disease or stroke. The pill can cause a rise in blood fat levels (cholesterol, LDL, and triglyceride levels). It can also cause problems with circulation and clotting. As the dose of estrogen and progestin has been decreased in newer pills, so has the risk decreased for these problems.

However, the risk for circulation and clotting problems is still quite high for women who smoke. Smoking causes the blood vessels to narrow, the walls of the vessels to thicken, and the blood to clot. That's why it is important for a woman to quit or reduce her smoking as much as possible. High $HbA_{1c}$ levels may also increase the chances of having blood-clotting problems.

It is important for a woman on the pill to have her $HbA_{1c}$, blood fats, and blood pressure checked *before and routinely after* starting the pill. If you have high blood pressure or high blood fats (hyperlipidemia), you may need to use a different method of contraception. Taking the pill when you have high blood pressure can increase the chance that eye or kidney disease will get worse. If you are concerned, speak to your doctor.

Side effects from the pill, such as weight gain, irritability, breast pain, or break-through bleeding are reasons many women stop taking the pill. These side effects are more common with progestin-only pills. If you experience any discomfort with taking any oral contraceptive, it is important to discuss other options with your provider. For the best results, keep your diabetes under reasonable control, take the pill as prescribed, and inform your health care provider when you have side effects. Of course, the pill does not provide you any protection against sexually transmitted diseases (STDs).

An Intrauterine Device (IUD) may be an attractive option for the woman who is past child bearing, is not likely to have any more children, and now has a single sex partner. In the past, women were discouraged from using the IUD because of the risk for pelvic infection or trauma to the uterine wall. The newer IUDs are considered to be far less likely to cause infection and undesired trauma. The IUD is an effective contraceptive method because it irritates the uterine wall making it difficult for the egg to get implanted. It may also be an effective choice because it does not affect blood glucose and blood fat levels.

Barrier methods such as the diaphragm or condoms with spermicidal foam or gels when used properly are effective methods that do not affect glucose control. The diaphragm is a rubber cap that the woman lubricates with a spermicidal gel and fits into her vagina and over her cervix before intercourse. It acts as a barrier to prevent sperm from entering the uterus. The uterus is where eggs are fertilized by the sperm. This is why it is called a barrier method of birth control. When used correctly, it can be up to 95% effective in preventing pregnancy.

Some women find the diaphragm awkward and difficult to use. They fear the loss of spontaneity in lovemaking. Because it can be inserted as much as an hour before intercourse, a little planning ahead will allow you to have some level of spontaneity. If you choose a diaphragm, it is important that your doctor fit it properly. Also, make sure he or she explains how to use it correctly. When women with diabetes use the diaphragm, they may have more yeast infections than women without diabetes.

Another barrier method of birth control is the condom, a thin membrane sheath that fits over the penis. There are larger ones made for women that cover the outer labia and fit into the vagina. A condom can be used effectively by itself, but it is even more effective when combined with a sperm-killing foam or vaginal gel. Statistics show that when the condom and foam are used together, they are up to 85% effective in preventing pregnancy. The major problem with barrier methods of birth control, such as the condom, is that they require some planning for use. They must be used every time intercourse occurs, and they must be used correctly. If not, they won't be effective. Condoms protect against STDs.

The use of implantable contraceptive agents, such as Norplant, and those requiring routine injection by your doctor, such as Depo-Provera, are other alternatives for women with diabetes. They will affect blood sugar levels. Norplant is a small capsule with medication in it that is placed under the skin on the arm. This capsule releases small amounts of the medication over a long period of time, approximately 5 years. It must be surgically removed. Depo-Provera must be injected by your doctor every three months. This is not the method of choice if you do not keep your appointments. Both methods need to be combined with a condom to prevent sexually transmitted diseases.

No matter what method you choose, be sure that it works for you, that you discuss side effects with your doctor, and that you inform your diabetes team about your contraceptive choice as this may affect your diabetes treatment program.

## Pregnancy

Women with type 1 and type 2 diabetes can have a healthy pregnancy and a healthy baby. This is especially true for women who keep blood sugar levels as close to normal as possible before and during the pregnancy. If you are contemplating having a child, you too can expect a healthy pregnancy. It is important for you to prepare for the pregnancy and to work with a team of professionals who are experienced and comfortable working with a woman with diabetes. Usually this team will consist of, at a minimum, a diabetes doctor, a high-risk obstetrician, a nurse educator, and a dietitian.

### Preparing for your pregnancy

Ideally, a woman should plan for her pregnancy 3–6 months before she gets pregnant. For some women, having to plan the pregnancy seems awkward and less romantic. But for a woman with diabetes, it is critical. The chance for birth defects and problems during pregnancy for the mother increases when diabetes is out of control or if there are other health problems that are not well managed. In order to reduce the risk for such problems, women with diabetes need to work with a team of professionals who can address all health issues and help them polish their diabetes self-management skills. Being a healthy mom greatly increases the chances of having a healthy baby!

To help you plan your pregnancy, use the following list. Every woman should have these areas evaluated before she gets pregnant. Your health care providers will help you determine when it is safe to become pregnant. If you can, shop around for a health care team that will work well with you.

Before getting pregnant, have the following evaluations done and discuss with your provider their influence on whether or when to get pregnant.

- **Eye evaluation.** Have a dilated eye exam with an ophthalmologist or an optometrist who is knowledgeable and experienced in managing diabetic retinopathy.
- **Blood pressure.** Pregnancy can cause blood pressure to rise. If uncontrolled, it can lead to problems with kidneys, heart, eyes, and the pregnancy itself.
- **HbA$_{1c}$ (overall blood glucose control).** Keeping HbA$_{1c}$ levels as close to normal as possible helps to provide a healthy environment for the baby to grow and develop.
- **Kidney test for protein.** The presence of protein may complicate the pregnancy.
- **Presence of hypoglycemia unawareness (inability to detect low blood sugar).** Diabetes providers work to adjust the treatment program, so that the woman is less at risk for experiencing severe low blood sugar levels.
- **Presence of heart disease or other circulatory problems.** Pregnancy can make these conditions worse and jeopardize the health of the woman and the baby. The doctor may advise against the pregnancy.
- **Breast exam, pelvic exam, and Pap smear.** It is important to have routine evaluations to ensure that the total body is as healthy as possible for the pregnancy.
- **Thyroid exam.** It is common for women with type 1 diabetes to have hypo- or hyperthyroid condition.

Members of the team will also want to review your diabetes management practices with you to ensure that you have the latest information and a program that is tailored to the needs of your body as it changes.

**Nutrition.** Your body's needs change during pregnancy. Work with a dietitian who can help you determine your caloric needs, your food choices, and the need for supplements. For instance, it is important for women to take folate (folic acid) supplements before getting pregnant to reduce the chance of having a baby with cleft palate or spina bifida. In addition, the dietitian can help you manage nausea and vomiting and ensure that you gain a healthy amount of weight. You'll need a different meal plan for breast-feeding, too.

**Diabetes medications.** Review insulin technique, sites, and adjustment practices. We don't know how oral diabetes pills affect the fetus, so the diabetes team will want to switch you to insulin well before you become pregnant.

**Self blood glucose monitoring.** Review technique and frequency. The frequency and timing may change at each trimester of the pregnancy and afterwards, especially if you are breastfeeding.

**Hypoglycemia.** What are your symptoms, frequency, severity, and treatment? Because your chances of experiencing low blood sugars increases during the first three months, it is important for you and your partner to know the signs and symptoms and to have a treatment plan in place.

**Hyperglycemia and sick day care.** Being pregnant does not increase your chances of getting sick. However, if you do get sick, it is important for you to know what to do, so that you can prevent ketoacidosis or very high blood sugars, which can put your baby at risk.

### During pregnancy

During pregnancy you will need to monitor blood glucose levels 4–10 times a day and to check your urine for ketones. You need to be prepared to make appropriate adjustments to your meal plan or insulin program, treat low blood sugar, and handle sick days. Working with a nurse and dietitian will help you learn these skills and more about how your diabetes will change during pregnancy.

Managing diabetes during pregnancy can be a challenge. The first three months are the most important to the development of the fetus. This is the time when the brain, nervous system, and body organs are developing. During this time, your blood sugar levels will change dramatically in response to hormone changes in your body and to morning sickness. Exhaustion and vomiting may further interfere with your ability to pay attention to your needs. Hormones released from the placenta during the second and third trimester make your body more resistant to insulin. You may be less sensitive to changes in blood sugar levels and to the warning signs of hypoglycemia. That's one of the reasons for needing to check your blood sugar more often.

Pregnancy can be an exciting and scary time. Learning and preparing as much as you can before getting pregnant will make a big difference for you, your family, and your baby.

## *Lactation*

Breastfeeding helps a new mother bond with her baby, regain her body shape, and enhance the baby's immune system, too. This can be a special and wonderful experience. It can also be challenging. Some infants take more time than others to learn how to latch onto the breast and to suckle, resulting in painful nipples, a frustrated mom, and an unhappy baby. Working with a supportive health care team will help you become confident and successful at breastfeeding your baby. Women with both type 1 and type 2 diabetes can breastfeed successfully.

Women who choose to breastfeed may experience low blood sugars that occur more often than before they were pregnant. The sugar levels drop as the baby feeds on the mother's milk. Some women report that their symptoms of low blood sugar change as well. It is possible to prevent frequent and severe low blood sugar through education and dietary counseling. Sugar or glucose tablets should be kept close by during feedings. You may need extra calories before, during, and after feeding the baby. Snacking or reducing the appropriate insulin will be important. Your insulin needs may be 25% lower than before becoming pregnant! This is particularly true to cover bedtime and night feedings.

The target ranges for your glucose control may be raised because you may experience low blood sugar in a more unpredictable fashion. It is also important to drink plenty of fluids and take in enough vitamins, minerals, and protein. Drinking a beverage each time you breastfeed is a good practice. Lactating women need 1,200–1,500 mg of calcium a day and enough calories to support both your and the baby's needs. Ask your dietitian about your nutritional needs and how to adjust your meal plan.

## *Menopause*

In a previous section, we described how a woman's comfort with intimacy and her sexual expression are related to her physical and emotional health. She is also influenced by society's ideas of what female sexuality should be. Menopause is yet another female process that is colored by society's expectations and perceptions. Calling it "the change" leaves many people with an image of a woman transforming into an odd, irrational being. There is nothing odd about menopause nor about the woman who is menopausal. It is a natural, normal transition in a woman's life. A transition that is revered and honored in many cultures. Your experience with menopause is influenced by how you feel about growing older and how you feel about passing from the reproductive phase of your life.

So what is menopause? Biologically it is the point at which a woman has not had a menstrual period for 12 months. Menopause is often a concern for women because it is associated with hot flashes, vaginal dryness, and other symptoms of estrogen deficiency. It marks the time when a women's risk for heart disease, osteoporosis, and other chronic diseases increases. Your body may feel like a stranger to you.

Natural menopause results from a progressive decline in estrogen production from the ovaries. Surgical menopause (hysterectomy) occurs when a woman's ovaries are removed, resulting in a dramatic decrease in estrogen. For the average woman, menopause occurs around the age of 51. The time before menopause is called *peri-menopause*. This is a time when our monthly cycle becomes more irregular and symptoms associated with menopause begin. The time after menopause is called *post-menopause.*

How you experience menopause is the result of many factors, including how you define your value as a woman and your thoughts and attitudes towards aging. The more that your define yourself based on your strengths, talents, and inner worth the more likely your are to accept the transitional symptoms associated with menopause. If you fear getting older and are resentful that your body is changing in ways that you are not receptive to, you are more likely to be less tolerant of this transition in your life.

Menopause is a convenient time to take stock of your health. It demands that a woman pay attention to her body. Changes occur that announce that her body is aging; skin is not as toned as before, weight begins to shift and settle more in the hips and belly. Things seem to move a little slower. She may become more aware of her sense of mortality, realizing that she is entering the last half of her life. This can be further intensified for women with diabetes because of the constant threat and reality of diabetic complications.

As estrogen production by the ovaries decreases, the lining of the vagina and bladder begins to thin, which can lead to vaginal dryness, pain with sexual activity, and urinary tract infections. Creams and gels can be used to restore moistness and tone. Hot flashes may occur as the levels of hormones fluctuate. Bones can become weaker because estrogen is needed to help maintain and stabilize bone strength. As less estrogen passes through the liver, the body produces less HDL (the good cholesterol), and the walls of the arteries can become less elastic and flexible. (More good reasons to eat whole foods and enjoy regular weight-bearing exercise to offset these changes.)

The frequency, intensity, and duration of hot flashes vary from person to person. Hot flashes contribute to sleep deprivation and fatigue. Some women do not experience any hot flashes, some have mild symptoms, and others suffer from severe symptoms. Hot flashes tend to persist for a couple of years. In rare cases, they can last 10 years or longer. There are some situations that aggravate the intensity of hot flashes, such as increased levels of psychological stress, hot and humid weather, confined spaces, alcohol, caffeine, and spicy foods. Hot flashes can be irritating and physically draining and negatively affect work, family, and social relationships. Medication, herbal preparations, and dietary phytoestrogens may help women manage the symptoms.

Menopause is a spiritual and emotional transition as well as a physical one. This normal process helps women make the transition from the age of childbearing and self-discovery to the age of wisdom and self-reflection. It is a time for women to reevaluate goals and priorities in their lives. Women experience menopause in different ways. Your experience will be influenced by your physical health, your attitudes, and your fears. Some women are elated about the freedom from periods, pregnancy, and need for contraception. Menopause signals that it is time to take time for introspection, inner growth, and spirituality. For other women, it is a time of grief and anxiety. Children may be leaving for college and creating their own lives. Others grieve the loss of being able to have a child. A woman's journey through menopause is personal. But it is a time to, in a real sense, give birth to herself.

In some cultures, menopausal and post-menopausal women are regarded as having power and insight of great value to the community. In our society, women are confronted with the attitude that menopause is a medical disease signaling a deficiency and an end to their sexuality and value. That's a limited and limiting perspective. You may want to take care not to get ensnared in it. Here's why.

Even though menopause marks the end of a woman's menstrual cycle, it does not mean that she is no longer a sexual being. We all know that a woman's worth and sexuality are not defined by her ability to have children. There are many women in their 60s, 70s, and 80s who remain strong, attractive, and vital. Look around! During this time of reflection, a woman comes into her own power. As author and teacher Caroline Myss points out, the post-menopausal woman tends to feel less bound to society's expectations and approval. She often feels freer to make choices and to engage in relationships that are mutually fulfilling. This can very well be a time of celebration like no other you've experienced!

## Experiences of diabetes during the peri-menopausal and menopausal years

When estrogen is present, your body is more sensitive to insulin. As levels of estrogen and progesterone fluctuate, you may experience wide swings in your blood sugars. Dr. Susan Love refers to menopause as puberty in reverse, wild with unpredictable swings in hormones and emotions. One month during the peri-menopausal years, the estrogen levels are high and the next month, they are low. Swings in hormones can cause difficulty sleeping, mood swings, and foggy thinking. These swings in hormones can play havoc with your blood sugar control. The subsequent high and low blood sugars can further aggravate the mood swings, foggy thinking, and sleeping problems.

Symptoms experienced during menopause can often be confused with the symptoms of low, and even high, blood sugars. Hot flashes, moodiness, and short-term memory loss can be mistaken as low blood sugar when, in fact, they are related to shifts in hormone levels. It is important for you to check your blood sugar before assuming that it is low and eating unnecessary calories. You may also see wide swings in glycemic control as your levels of hormones change, which can be further complicated by inadequate sleep.

During menopause, women often report low blood sugars that are stronger and more frequent, especially during the middle of the night. Sleep is often disrupted by hot flashes and night sweats. Controlling diabetes can difficult, just as it is during adolescence. Teenagers also experience unpredictable swings in blood sugar related to rapidly fluctuating hormone levels. Dealing with the feelings of moodiness and fatigue or with the unpredictability of hot flashes and fluctuations in blood sugar can leave a woman feeling isolated and frustrated. Some women find that their body is more resistant to insulin and that their blood sugars are much higher, requiring increases in their medication or a need to start new medication. This is particularly true if a woman gains weight or reduces her level of activity during the menopausal years.

As you move through the menopause period, levels of estrogen and progesterone permanently decrease and the body becomes less resistant to insulin. Hypoglycemia, (low blood sugars) can occur. You may need to decrease the dose of your diabetes medications. Talk with your health care provider about this.

The effects of vaginal dryness and changes in the bladder that occur as a result of estrogen deficiency can be made worse by persistent high blood sugars. You might be more susceptible to vaginal yeast infections and urinary tract infections. Honest discussions with your health care providers are important so that you get the right treatment. Prompt treatment of vaginal and urinary tract infections are important for many reasons because infections can further disrupt your blood sugar balance.

If these experiences sound familiar to you, we hope that you take comfort in knowing that you are not alone. Moving through this transition, which can take months to a few years, can be challenging. Discussing the issues honestly with good listeners like friends, family, and health care providers is one approach to keep in mind. If you haven't already, this may be the time that you see a gynecologist regularly to work with you and your diabetes team. Gynecologists and their teams are equipped with tips and strategies for getting through the tough hot flashes and dealing with changes in your sex life and sex drive that may result from vaginal dryness and thinning of the vaginal tissues. They keep up with the literature and science, so they are more likely to have an array of interventions—nutritional, lifestyle, and other approaches—that might meet your needs.

Your diabetes treatment program probably also needs attention. It might be time to visit your diabetes team to explore the possibility of changing your medication program. There are more types of oral medications and insulin programs now available that might address the changing needs of your body. Reviewing your meal plan strategies and choices may provide you with some different ideas and information you need to promote diabetes control as well as determine how your nutritional needs are changing.

The media are full of suggestions and advice as to what supplements to use and what foods to eat. The amount of information can be overwhelming. Working with a dietitian who knows the science and can decipher what is right for you might save you time and a lot of frustration. During the periods of time when the blood sugars are most challenging, some women have found it helpful to simplify their life by getting back on a tighter schedule. This means that they try to reduce the number of factors that affect their blood sugar levels, so that they can get a better idea about where to make changes.

> *Louisa has type 2 diabetes. After consulting with her diabetes team, she went back to following her meal plan as closely as possible and focused on taking her medications at a set time every day. This allowed her and her doctor to look at the effects of fluctuating hormones on her blood sugar without the "noise" of other factors getting in the way.*

As stated earlier, this is a time that your body calls for attention. Getting adequate sleep and trying relaxation techniques to help balance the effects of emotional and physical stress may help you. Pushing the limit (as women often do!) usually complicates diabetes control and the symptoms of hot flashes, irritability, moodiness, and our ability to concentrate. So, take a nap when you need to (if you can) and remember to breathe deeply and slowly as often as you can! As Jesse, a woman with type 1 diabetes stated, "My best friend is my breath. It is always with me. When I am troubled, scared, and bothered, breathing deeply allows me to get back into my body, get centered, and feel energized."

Humor and patience are valuable when going through transitions that are unpredictable like menopause. If you find yourself disgusted or frustrated, you might want to consider an approach like Jordan's, a 16 year old with type 1 diabetes. In response to widely fluctuating blood sugars resulting from puberty, she would exclaim

"It must be those HORMS!" What a perfect expression to capture our sense of powerlessness over this situation. Sometimes our body rules! This humor and lighthearted approach is also refreshing and healthy! It allowed her to observe the changes that were sometimes outside of her control without anger, shame, and guilt. It allowed her to be open to suggestions for improvement and to preserve the energy she needed to figure out what to do next. If you are going through a challenging time, try to be gentle and not critical of yourself.

If you believe that menopause is a journey that is truly spiritual, emotional, and physical, then you might find comfort in knowing that through this transition you can encounter new aspects of yourself and discover new interests, hidden talents, or desires. Be open to the new sides of yourself that may emerge. Be willing to be surprised. In the process, consider reaching out and talking to other women, with and without diabetes, who are also experiencing or have gone through this transition. You will most likely find that you are not alone in your experience. This circle of wisdom might shed some light about how you can reshape your life to fit your needs and desires in ways you never thought possible.

*For Candace, a woman with type 2 diabetes, menopause has interfered with changes in blood sugar and overall energy. "Over the last three months my blood sugar was acting very strange. Sometimes I have even had a low sugar—that is unusual for me! Other times, it is high and I am feeling crabby. This is all worse when I am stressed out about work. My doctor told me that it might be related to menopause. Wow! I guess there is nothing for me to do but accept it. I can't change my biological clock. This is very frustrating.*

*My symptoms of low blood sugar are very similar to having a hot flash. I now have to check my blood sugar when the symptoms occur to be sure which one it may be. It can be a hassle. My doctor and I are considering estrogen replacement therapy. My sister who is five years older than me told me that yoga helped her. I might try that as well."*

Menopausal changes in hormone levels can disrupt glucose control and make the body more sensitive to insulin. There are many options for dealing with the symptoms of menopause. Patience and being gentle to yourself during this time of transition is important. Remember it's those HORMS!

## Managing Menopausal Health

Like many things in medicine, the viewpoints on how to treat menopause are polarized. One view is that menopause is a deficiency state that should be managed medically to treat symptoms and prevent disease. Another view is that it is a normal life passage that should not be overmedicated. The reality is that some menopausal symptoms are disruptive, and they can be relieved by medications. The other reality is that as a woman goes through menopause, her production of estrogen is dramatically reduced, which can increase her risk for heart disease, osteoporosis, and dementia. Therefore, some women, especially those at risk, may benefit from medications to help in their efforts to prevent and manage these disease states. (A more detailed description of the risk factors for heart disease, osteoporosis, and breast cancer follows later in this chapter.)

Keep in mind the key phrase "at risk." Not all women carry the same risk. For some the effects of estrogen deficiency are more dramatic than for others. For example, women having a hysterectomy have a sudden drop in estrogen levels. They might experience symptoms more dramatically than a woman who goes through menopause naturally, where there is a gradual loss in estrogen. A woman must sit down and evaluate her personal health profile to determine whether she is more or less at risk. If her risk is high, preventive medical approaches may be worth her while if the pros outweigh the cons. If her risk is low, she might be able to use less aggressive preventive approaches.

*Nora is a 53-year-old woman with type 2 diabetes. She is now post-menopausal. Having diabetes and being menopausal are 2 risk factors for heart disease. She is trying to determine with her doctor whether or not to take medication to reduce her risk for heart disease and osteoporosis. Her father had a heart attack at the age of 63. Her lipids are elevated. Her bone density scan revealed that she has osteopenia (low bone mass). Her grandmother and mother both lost height as they aged and suffered from spinal fractures. Nora and her doctor decided that she is at high risk for developing osteoporosis and heart disease. Hormone therapy may be a wise choice for her along with a low-fat meal plan and an activity program that is aerobic and includes weight-bearing exercise.*

*Morie is a 54-year-old woman with type 2 diabetes. She also is postmenopausal. Her bone mass is normal. Her grandmother did suffer from a hip fracture at the age of 88 and her mother has been diagnosed with osteoporosis. Heart disease is a problem in her family. Her lipids are slightly elevated but not alarming. She is aware that because she has diabetes, she is at risk for heart disease and that, although she does not have a problem with osteoporosis at this time, it might become an issue as she ages. So she and her doctor agreed to begin a prevention plan that relies on nutritional changes, aerobic and weight-bearing exercise, and adequate nutritional supplements. They agree that close monitoring of markers of heart and bone disease is important to help determine whether she'll need medication in the future.*

"Ah," you say, "What about my grandmother? She lived to the ripe old age of 78 without worrying about menopause!" While it is true that many of our grandmothers lived long lives, it is also true that their lifestyle, the types of stresses, and the environmental exposures were very different. For instance, their lifestyle involved more physical labor (hard work) and fewer processed foods. It is also possible that our mothers or grandmothers did suffer from menopausal symptoms but did not discuss them. In the past, it was less common for women to express problems with their emotional and physical health than it is today. So for these reasons, and others, be cautious when referring to your grandmother's experiences.

In deciding whether or not hormone replacement therapy is for you, it is important to look at all the pieces of the puzzle to get the big picture of your risk profile. In determining which options are best for you, you might want to take into account the points outlined here and discuss them with your health care provider.

- genetic make-up and family history: health problems and experiences with side effects of medications or interventions
- your past and current lifestyle: nutritional practices, activity levels and types of activity, and relaxation methods and practices
- external stresses and how you handle them
- your clinical profile: weight, bone density, lipids, blood pressure, etc.
- attitude: about taking care of yourself, about prevention, about your body, etc.

The goal in health care is to maximize the quality of your life as you age, so that you are as strong and vital as you can be. The years right before, during, and after menopause—40s through 70s—is a time that many women actively seek ways to reduce their risk for the health problems we've just discussed. We are calling you into action—no matter what age you are—to get you motivated to prevent or minimize any health problems.

*Myra has diabetes and is now transitioning through menopause. "I am just beginning to deal with menopause. Up until seven months ago, I thought that I had come to terms with dealing with diabetes. I was able to manage the routine; you know, treat the high and low blood sugars and take my insulin on time. Besides that, I have just realized that because I have diabetes, my chances for developing heart disease is even greater! My father and uncle died of heart attacks in their early sixties. I get anxious knowing that I am getting to that age. I have to pay closer attention to my blood fats and fit exercise in. Sometimes I wonder, why me?"*

Having to confront her mortality and the potential for more health problems has Myra feeling vulnerable, scared, and resentful. The positive thing is that she isn't running away from it. She's exercising more and getting her health care provider's help to bring the blood fat levels down. Her feelings are valid and honest. Her fear is real. And she isn't alone. It is common for a woman facing menopause to stop and reflect on the meaning of her life. Diabetes increases her risk for many health problems. Understanding this has now motivated her to make some lifestyle change. There are things that she can do to reduce the chances of her developing heart problems. What she needs to do to take care of her diabetes is often the same thing she needs to care for herself in general. Healthy living is healthy living.

## Estrogen and Hormone Replacement Therapy

Hormone replacement therapy (HRT) is a hot topic in women's health. Many women use HRT to alleviate menopausal symptoms such as hot flashes and vaginal dryness. HRT is approved for the prevention of osteoporosis and is believed to reduce a woman's risk for heart disease, colon cancer, dementia, and possibly Alzheimer's disease. Many women are drawn to HRT by the possibilities of getting smoother, younger looking skin, increased vitality, and improved sexual function. Despite the perceived benefits of HRT, there is a great deal of controversy about it. Why? There is concern about an increased risk for some types of breast and uterine cancer. In addition, many of the reported benefits are based on population-based studies, observational studies as opposed to randomized, intervention studies. Observational studies are not as scientifically rigorous as intervention studies, which leaves many questions unanswered.

## Taking hormone replacement therapy

There are many different preparations of estrogen and progestin (the synthetic form of progesterone). Each acts differently in the body according to the type and routes of administration and your body chemistry. Estrogen replacement therapy (ERT) refers to treatment with estrogen alone, which is only appropriate for women without a uterus. HRT refers to the combination of estrogen and progestin, which is the treatment for women with a uterus. The most common brands of estrogen used are Premarin for ERT, and Prempro is used for HRT. Most major studies conducted in the United States have used these preparations.

There are three different ways to take estrogen for ERT.

- **Oral.** Oral estrogen can be taken alone if you do not have a uterus. This is called unopposed estrogen. There are different types of estrogens: conjugated equine estrogen (CEE); natural estrogen (such as estradiol); synthetic estrogen (ethinyl estradiol). If you do have a uterus, you will need to take a combination of estrogen and progestin. Oral estrogen has the greatest benefit on blood lipid levels. This is felt to be due to its effect on cholesterol metabolism in the liver.

- **Vaginal cream.** Estrogen applied to the vagina in the form of vaginal creams, or the estrogen ring, alleviate menopausal changes that affect the female genitals, such as vaginal dryness, thinning of the delicate lining of the vagina, and leaking of urine (incontinence). Because this form of estrogen is neither absorbed into the bloodstream in significant amounts nor passed through the liver, it is not effective on blood lipid levels. Nor is it helpful in promoting stronger bones or insulin sensitivity.

- **Patch.** The estrogen patch also appears to be helpful in alleviating menopausal symptoms, yet may have a limited effect on lipids because it doesn't pass through the liver.

HRT is taken in pill form in different combinations. Progestins are used in combination with estrogen to protect the uterus from precancerous changes and uterine cancer. The most common types used in the U.S. are MPA (Provera) and micronized progesterone (natural progesterone), in a pill called Prometrium.

You can take progestin and estrogen in one of two ways: in continuous combined therapy or cyclical therapy by taking the progestin during part of the month.

- Continuous combined therapy: Both estrogen and progestin are taken every day. They can be combined in one pill. This approach helps to eliminate the problem of monthly bleeding, yet may cause irregular spotting, bloating, and some emotional side effects such as irritability and mood swings.
- Cyclic HRT: Estrogen is taken every day and progestin is added for 10–14 days of the month. This will cause a woman to resume vaginal bleeding every month.

For a list of different estrogen and progestin preparations and doses see Table 6-1 on page 168.

Sometimes the usual estrogen dose of 0.625 mg per day is not enough to alleviate all of the symptoms experienced during menopause. Occasionally the dose can be increased for short periods of time. Or other ways can be tried to cope with symptoms (avoiding triggers, relaxation, etc.). But more than likely your physician will not increase the dose in order to protect you from the side effects. To reap the most benefit from HRT you will need to take it for a long time. This is especially true for the prevention of osteoporosis and heart disease. When you stop taking HRT, you will gradually lose the benefits.

## Advantages of HRT

**Heart.** Many observational studies have shown that HRT reduces a woman's risk for heart disease, heart attacks, and related deaths. The positive effect of HRT is related to its beneficial effect on lipids (blood fats) and non-lipid factors such as its ability to improve clotting factors and to dilate arteries.

**Lipid effects.** Both estrogen and hormone replacement therapies have positive and negative effects on blood lipids.

Positive effects on lipids include

- an increase in the body's production of HDL, the good cholesterol
- a decrease in the body's production of LDL, the bad cholesterol, which accumulates in blood vessel walls
- a decrease in total cholesterol

When used alone, estrogen has a greater beneficial effect than when it is combined with progestin. This means that women on HRT, the combination of progestin and estrogen, may experience a lesser increase in HDL and smaller decrease in LDL levels.

An undesirable side effect of estrogen and hormone replacement therapy is that it causes a rise in triglycerides. This may be particularly problematic for women with type 2 diabetes or with high levels of triglycerides.

There are no long-term studies looking at the effects of hormone replacement therapy in women with diabetes. It is important, if you have started on HRT, that you have your lipids (total cholesterol, LDL, HDL and triglycerides) checked before and regularly after starting therapy. If you have high triglycerides, it might be prudent for you not to take HRT because the level may only go higher.

**Blood vessel effects.** Hormone replacement therapy

- helps dilate blood vessels and increases blood flow
- helps keep blood vessels flexible
- decreases fibrinogen and other factors related to clotting

Estrogen alone has been shown to help decrease factors that promote excessive clotting and heart disease. There have been no large, long-term studies looking at the effects of estrogen on clotting in women with diabetes. Based on what is known about the positive effects of hormone replacement therapy on blood vessels, many experts believe that it can be valuable for women with diabetes.

## Hormone replacement therapy and diabetes

Studies suggest that some preparations of estrogen promote insulin sensitivity, which may in turn lead to a lowering of blood sugars. However, the combination of estrogen and progestin does not seem to affect glucose control. It is unknown whether the use of the forms of progesterone will result in an improvement or worsening of blood sugar control.

Population-based studies show that women who have diabetes may not respond as well to HRT as women who don't have diabetes. HDL levels increase but not as much. Triglycerides tend to rise more than they do in women without diabetes. Of the studies done in women with diabetes taking estrogen, however, it appears that estrogen is effective in improving lipid levels.

In summary, studies suggest that estrogen is helpful in improving the ability of the blood vessel to dilate and be flexible, raising HDL, and lowering LDL levels. Estrogen may also lower blood glucose levels and decrease blood-clotting factors. The effects of HRT on these variables in women with diabetes are unknown. Worsening of high triglyceride levels is a possible side effect of HRT for women with diabetes. Long-term clinical trials looking at the effects of ERT or HRT on the rate of heart attacks or cardiac related death in women with diabetes are needed.

The Women's Health Initiative, a large randomized clinical trial, is currently under way to compare the effect of nutrition and hormone replacement therapy on reducing a woman's risk for heart disease. Because of its size, it will include women with diabetes and hopefully provide us with more insights about their special needs.

# Studies of the Effect of HRT on Heart Disease

Decisions about ERT and HRT use to prevent heart disease can be guided by the results of 3 major studies looking at the effect of hormone replacement therapy on heart disease. The Nurse's Health Study and PEPI trial are observational studies. The HERS study is a randomized, clinical trail. As we have discussed before, observational studies show that HRT use is associated with a lower risk for heart disease. These studies do not prove that HRT use is responsible for the low risk. In fact, women who choose to take HRT tend to have fewer risk factors for heart disease. Their lower risk for heart disease may just be the result of their healthier lifestyle and not due to HRT use at all.

### Nurses Health Study

This was a population-based study of more than 121,000 nurses who were followed for many years. Women lived their life as they normally would. They were asked to complete a survey that questioned them about their health habits, health problems, lifestyle, and medications.

The findings showed that women currently taking HRT had a higher HDL than women who used HRT in the past or who never used it. Current HRT users were likely to have fewer heart attacks and deaths related to heart disease than past users. Estrogen treatment alone was more effective in raising HDL and lowering LDL and total cholesterol than the combination of estrogen and progestin. These results suggest that the addition of progestin blunts the positive effects of estrogen on the heart.

### HERS—Heart Estrogen/Progestin Replacement Study

This study looked at more than 2,700 women with pre-existing heart disease and compared the effects of HRT (Prempro) versus placebo on reducing heart attacks and cardiac-related deaths. This was a randomized clinical trial that lasted 4 years. It showed that there was no benefit of HRT in women with pre-existing coronary heart disease. In fact, during the first year, women on HRT experienced more heart attacks than women on placebo. Experts continue to debate what caused the results. There is a great deal of concern that the type of progestin used may have been the culprit. More and more physicians are now considering the use of micronized progesterone (Prometrium) because it has fewer side effects.

As a result of this study, the American Heart Association and the American College of Cardiology caution against starting HRT in women with pre-existing heart disease. It is considered safe for women already taking HRT to continue it, however, even if they have heart disease.

### PEPI—Postmenopausal Estrogen and Progestin Intervention Trial

This 3-year study randomized 875 women aged 45–64 years into 1 of 5 different treatment groups: a placebo pill, estrogen, or different combinations of HRT. It was designed to look at the effects of these drugs on blood-fat levels. Results showed that women taking ERT or HRT had an increase in HDL, decrease in LDL, a decrease cholesterol, and an increase in triglycerides. When comparing HRT combinations to ERT, they found that HDL increased in women taking HRT but less than in women who took estrogen alone. They also found that HDL levels were slightly higher in women who took Prometrium when compared to women who took Prempro.

Researchers concluded that both ERT and HRT are effective in improving the lipid profile of women. They noted that estrogen alone was more powerful in increasing HDL cholesterol than any HRT preparation.

## Osteoporosis

Many observational studies have shown that oral ERT and HRT prevents or halts the progression of bone loss after menopause. It has been shown to increase bone density slightly. As a result, the risk for fractures of the spine and possibly of the hip may be reduced.

Estrogen helps to promote strong bones because it enhances vitamin D absorption, which in turn is important for the absorption of calcium. It helps to reduce the rate of bone loss. Without estrogen, the body loses bone mass, increasing a woman's risk for fractures.

While looking at the factors that were related to a risk for heart disease, researchers from the Framingham Heart Study also looked at the relationship between HRT use and osteoporosis. They noted that women who took hormones seemed to have fewer hip fractures and less osteoporosis than women who did not. Supplements of calcium and vitamin D are important for strengthening bones. Daily calcium intake of at least 1,000 mg a day and 400–800 IU of vitamin D a day is recommended for all women. (Vaginal creams or estrogen patches are not helpful in preventing osteoporosis.)

If osteoporosis is severe, estrogen can be combined with Fosamax (a drug to strengthen bones) to achieve greater increases in bone density. Estrogen should not be combined with Evista (another drug which can prevent bone loss), because they may compete with each other in the bone tissue and increase the risk for blood clots to unacceptable levels.

## Side Effects

Women differ in their response to hormone therapy. It is important to let your health care provider know if you are experiencing any difficulty. Side effects of HRT include breast tenderness and soreness, nausea, headaches, heavy bleeding, leg cramps, abdominal fullness, fluid retention, irritability, mood swings, and acne. Women with migraines may experience an increase in headaches. HRT can also cause an increase in gallstone problems. Many of these side effects are generally associated with oral estrogen or estrogen and progestin preparations. Skin patches and vaginal forms of estrogen do not carry the same degree of side effects.

## What about the long term risks?

There are 3 major long-term health problems associated with taking ERT or HRT: breast cancer, uterine cancer, and deep vein blood clots.

**Breast Cancer.** Estrogen signals many cells in the body to "grow and divide." Long-term exposure to this message stimulates the growth of abnormal cells that may eventually become cancerous. The breast and uterus are both sensitive to this message. HRT has been associated with a 30–50% increased risk for types of breast cancer that are dependent on estrogen to grow. At this time, HRT use does not appear to be related to an increased risk for any other type of breast cancer.

Many observational studies have looked at the relationship between HRT and breast cancer. The risk for breast cancer in a woman on hormones depends on her age and how long she takes hormones. In the Nurse's Health Study, researchers found that women between the ages of 65 and 69 who were currently taking HRT experienced a 71% increased risk for breast cancer as compared to a 54% increased risk for women between the age of 55 and 59.

Overall, the data from multiple studies suggest that taking HRT for more than 5 years increases the average woman's risk of breast cancer by 30%. To put this in perspective, 12 out of 100 women not taking HRT will experience breast cancer, while 18 out of 100 women on HRT will. The risk increases more after 10 years of continued use and even more so after 15. The longer the use, the greater the risk.

A woman's risk is also linked with current use. In the Iowa Women's Health Study, published in 1999, an increased risk of breast cancer was observed in women who were current users of HRT. This finding is consistent with other studies. A woman's risk for breast cancer decreases after she stops taking ERT or HRT.

Some researchers have found an increased trend for breast cancer in women who consume one or more drinks of alcohol a day. This has lead to the idea that alcohol consumption increases estrogen levels in women and this is problematic especially for women who are current hormone users. Other studies suggest that women who gain weight while on hormones may also be more at risk than women whose weight is stable.

Estrogen is generally not considered an option for women with a personal or family history of breast cancer. This is an issue of great debate and concern in the medical community. In order to address this issue, we need large randomized studies looking at the effects of HRT on women who have survived breast cancer or who have a high risk for breast cancer.

**Uterine cancer.** If a woman does not have a uterus, she can take estrogen therapy without progestin, such as estradiol, estraderm, or equine estrogen (Premarin). As estrogen gives the body a "grow and divide" message, progestin stops this message in the breast. When taken alone, estrogen can cause the lining of the uterus to thicken and develop abnormal cells, which can lead to uterine cancer. The additional progestin prevents this process. In the 1970s and 1980s, studies showed that when estrogen was used alone in women with a uterus, the risk for uterine cancer increased sixfold. Therefore, if a woman has her uterus, she will need to take progestin to oppose the effects of estrogen and reduce the risk for developing uterine (endometrial) cancer.

**Risk for blood clots.** In the past, the dose of estrogen used in HRT regimens and oral contraceptives was much higher than it is today. These higher doses of estrogen often interfered with the anti-clotting factors in the blood and resulted in more blood clots in the legs and lungs as well as strokes. The risk for blood clots in the leg and lungs still exist, but it is much lower than in the past. The risk for experiencing blood clots increases with age, with a previous history of blood clots, and during long periods of immobility or inactivity.

Estrogen therapy is not appropriate for women with a history of severe clotting disorders. The use of transdermal patches or vaginal cream does not tend to affect the body's clotting ability and may be a treatment option for women with clotting disorders.

## Taking Hormone Replacement Therapy

Before starting HRT, it is important for you to have a thorough check-up. This exam should include an assessment of your risk for developing heart disease, osteoporosis, and breast and uterine cancer, a breast exam, a mammogram, a pelvic exam, and Pap smear; blood work to check your liver function, thyroid function, lipid levels,

| TABLE 6-1 | | |
|---|---|---|
| Preparation | Side Effects and Risks | Benefits |
| Estrogen Therapy Premarin Estratab Estrace Ogen, Ortho-Est | Increased risk of uterine cancer (when taken without progestin); breast cancer, gallbladder disease, deep-vein blood clots, and increased triglycerides | Relieves symptoms Increases bone mass Raises HDL, lowers LDL |
| Progestin Therapy Provera Prometrium | Cyclic progestin causes menstrual bleeding | Decreases risk of uterine cancer, slightly reduced the beneficial effect on lipids |

| TABLE 6-1 *(Continued)* | | |
|---|---|---|
| **Preparation** | **Side Effects and Risks** | **Benefits** |
| *Combination Therapy* | Carries same risk as estrogen therapy except for uterine cancer (and possibly breast cancer). | Relieves symptoms Increases bone mass Raises HDL, lowers LDL, yet to a lesser degree than estrogen alone Decreases risk of uterine cancer |
| Prempro | Cyclic progestin causes menstrual bleeding | |
| Premphase | Continuous combined HRT causes irregular bleeding | |
| Estratest | | |
| *Patches* Estraderm FemPatch Combipath | Skin allergies | Relieves vaginal dryness and hot flashes Reduces risk of osteoporosis |
| *Vaginal Creams* Estrace cream Premarin cream Ortho Dienestrol cream | May increase risk for uterine cancer | Helps prevent urinary tract infections |
| *Other Source* Estring (vaginal ring) | May be expelled | Relieves vaginal dryness May prevent urinary tract infections |

calcium levels, and hemoglobin $A_{1c}$. The benefits and risks of any therapy like HRT are individual and can be altered by your own medical history and your family history. Decisions about treatment are related to your attitude about the health problem and the proposed treatment as well as your providers' attitudes It is important to explore and discuss these issue as you determine what is best for you.

## Alternative therapies for managing menopausal health

While many women choose HRT to relieve the discomforts of menopause, other women choose alternative medications and herbal therapies. Increasingly, women are drawn to "natural" alternatives like soy products and herbs that have been used by women in many countries.

### Soy

Soy is a phytoestrogen, a natural plant estrogen. It appears that soy reduces the frequency and severity of hot flashes about half as well as hormone therapy. Soy's effect on osteoporosis and heart disease is not clearly known yet, but initial results from observational studies are promising. Data suggests that consuming foods rich in phytoestrogens does appear to have a weak estrogen-like effect on preventing bone loss. Some studies have shown that 47 grams of soy protein taken on a daily basis decreases LDL cholesterol, decreases triglycerides, and does not increase HDL. Study results on the effects of soy on breast cancer are conflicting. Experts caution women not to draw any conclusions at this time because no clinical trial looking at this has been done.

Phytoestrogens attracted interest in this culture when it was realized that women in Japan did not suffer from hot flashes or other symptoms of menopause. It is believed that this is related to the fact that Japanese women consume a diet rich in soy products. However, it appears that nutrition and lifestyle factors may only account for some of the difference. Researchers have discovered that women from other cultures also do not experience menopausal symptoms. Cultural beliefs influence whether a woman experiences the changes in her body as negative or positive. If a woman experiences them as negative, she is more likely to be bothered by them. Some cultures do not have words in their vocabulary like "hot flash," so are less likely to report such problems. There also may be biological reasons for differences. Women of different cultures may physically react differently to the changes in hormone levels.

Soybeans and flaxseed are abundant sources of phytoestrogens. To obtain an effective dose, a woman may need to consume at least 40 grams of a substance that contains 75 mg of phytoestrogens. This is referred to as total isoflavone content on the label. If you are going to take flaxseed oil or capsules instead of grinding or cooking the flax seed, be sure it is fresh. Rancid oil is not good for you.

It appears that pills and supplements are not as effective in reducing hot flashes as foods containing soy protein with phytoestrogens. Experts also caution women that the capsules found in stores are not monitored by the FDA and may contain levels that are less or more than is considered effective. Keep in mind that randomized studies of large numbers of women to evaluate the effectiveness of soy have not been done yet. Research on the safety and effectiveness of these therapies continues.

**Nutrition**

If you are not eating vegetables and greens, then you are missing out on nature's powerhouse of vitamins and minerals meant just for you. Women who eat dark green vegetables, such as kale, collard greens, spinach, and Swiss chard, benefit greatly. And if you want to take a note from grandmother, try dandelion greens and nettles. It's not likely that you'll be gathering these in the field, but you can buy them fresh, dried, or preserved in an alcohol tincture at the local health food store or whole foods market. You might try "greening" your diet and see how you feel.

Your adrenal glands are called on during menopause to produce estrogen because the ovaries stop producing it. Try to move away from white flour and white sugar and to eat more whole grains. What you eat does make a difference to your whole body, not just your diabetes!

### Herbs

Because of a growing interest in natural remedies for women's conditions, research studies are now being done to determine the benefits of certain herbs on women's health. Those results are not in yet, so the herbs we discuss here have been used for hundreds of years in other cultures, and in Europe they are used routinely to help women because they have a milder affect on the body than ERT or HRT. The herbs for possible use with menopausal symptoms are chastetree berry, garden sage, motherwort, black cohosh, ginseng, and dong quai. You can find herbs in several forms: fresh, as a tea, as an alcohol tincture, or in capsules.

As you should do before you take any medication, discuss the potential benefits and side effects of the herb with a health professional, preferably one who is knowledgeable about herbs and their effects on body chemistry. If you want to find a qualified herbalist or traditional Chinese practitioner, check the Resources at the end of this chapter for organizations that can help you. If you are taking medication, find out how the herb you want to try will interact with it before you try it.

Chastetree berry is an herb that has been used by women throughout the ages. It has a gentle effect that balances a woman's system, affecting hormones to tone down PMS symptoms and cramps and ease the transition of menopause. Its action is slow and most women only notice its effect after several months. There are no reported side effects of using it.

Garden sage is a common herb, but it has other uses than just flavoring the turkey dressing at Thanksgiving. It, too, balances a woman's system. It is believed to ease night sweats in menopause as well as emotional swings. It strengthens the liver and aids digestion. A cup of sage tea may be what you need on a chaotic day. Don't use it too much, however, because it can be too drying to mucous membranes in mouth and vagina, and the essential oils in it can accumulate in the kidneys and liver.

Motherwort is said to ease heart palpitations and hot flashes. It is high in calcium and may help tone the heart and uterus and help you sleep. It also helps restore tone and moisture to the vagina. If you are experiencing menstrual flooding, this herb may make it worse, so don't take it at those times.

Black Cohosh is a strong herb that was used by American Indians for common menopausal symptoms. Black cohosh has a beneficial effect on the heart and blood vessels and nourishes the adrenal glands. Do not use black cohosh if you are pregnant or have menstrual flooding. It can cause side effects, most particularly headache or nausea. Get advice from a health care professional about the best way to use this herb.

Ginseng has been used by the Chinese and American Indians to help regulate a woman's symptoms during her cycles and to give her more energy. Research done in the U.S. in the past 50 years shows that ginseng has a beneficial effect on the heart, lowering blood pressure and cholesterol levels. It is believed to slow aging with antioxidants. Don't use ginseng if you have a fever or are nervous and jittery. Good quality ginseng is expensive, so if you find a bargain brand, be aware that it probably contains little ginseng.

Dong quai has been used in China for thousands of years as a blood tonic. This herb affects the body as estrogen does to ease hot flashes, night sweats, and other menopausal symptoms. It contains calcium, too. Don't take it during a period or with a fever. Dong quai also boosts your immune system and aids in circulation.

Herbs can be helpful for a woman, but you need to know how to use them correctly to get the benefits. Your body chemistry is unique and herbs can interact with it very powerfully. It is best to discuss any herbs you want to use with a registered dietitian or qualified herbalist who is trained to evaluate the effect the herbs will likely have on you.

### Vitamins and minerals

As we say elsewhere in this book, you should be getting 1,200–1,500 mg of calcium a day and about 400–800 IU of vitamin D. This helps keep your bones strong. Vitamin E is considered the anti-aging and help-for-menopausal-symptoms vitamin. Many researchers are now recommending a daily intake of 400–800 IUs of vitamin E. In addition, if you find that mood swings affect you and you're under a lot of stress, try B-complex vitamins. You can get them from eating whole grains and other foods, but the body does not store them, and you use them up pretty quickly under stress.

Alternative health practices, like the ones we have discussed here, are only just being examined by the research community to determine what effects, interactions, and uses will be scientifically proven effective and thus best to use.

## Breast Health

Breast cancer is getting a lot of media attention in the U.S. Many women believe that it is the number one threat to their health. Fear and misperceptions about the risks and about treatments are motivating women to follow many treatments that have not yet been proven. The reality is that fewer women are diagnosed or die of breast cancer than heart disease. Heart disease continues to be the leading cause of death in women. If a woman lives to the age of 80, she has a 1 in 9 chance in having breast cancer and a 1 in 3 chance of developing heart disease.

Many studies are under way to determine the causes and cures for breast cancer. What researchers know and agree upon is that early detection and treatment is critical for better prognosis. We want to be sure that you keep your breast health in mind as part of your total health package.

Most breast tumors are slow growing. Experts believe that from the time that the cancer starts, it takes 7–10 years before it is visible on a mammogram. Knowing your risk and engaging in good breast health practices may increase your chances of early detection and cure.

### How do I know whether I am at risk?

Several factors put a woman at risk for breast cancer. Yet, 70% of the women who develop breast cancer do not appear to have any of these risk factors. There may be a genetic link. Evidence also suggests that obesity and the use of drugs containing hormones may increase a woman's risk. In *Dr. Susan Love's Breast Book*, Dr. Love reports studies that suggest the risk for breast cancer increases when a women is exposed to alcohol, radiation, and high-fat diets during her youth, the time between her first period and the time of her first pregnancy. It appears that as breast tissue is developing, it is very sensitive to carcinogens. If this proves to be true, it may mean that our risk for breast cancer is laid out for us in our early years and that the chance of developing breast cancer increases the more exposure we have to other factors as we age.

The known risk factors are

- **Age.** As we get older, the risk for breast cancer increases.
- **Family history.** Having a first-degree relative (a mother or sister) with breast cancer increases your risk. However, not all breast cancers are related to family history. Family history of ovarian, uterine, colon, or prostate cancer has been linked to an increased risk for breast cancer.
- **Personal history.** Having a previous diagnosis of atypical breast disease may indicate that you have a risk that is higher than normal. Your risk is increased if you have had ovarian, uterine, colon, or previous breast cancer.
- **Radiation exposure.** Exposure to radiation, especially in younger women increases the risk for breast cancer.

It is believed that the risk for breast cancer is also related to a woman's exposure to her own estrogen. Estrogen gives the breast tissue a grow and divide message. The more exposure to this message or to outside sources of estrogen, the greater the chances are of developing abnormal cells. The longer the exposure, the greater the risk. So women with the following characteristics are at increased risk

- early menstrual cycle, starting before the age of 12
- late menopause, experienced after the age of 55
- late childbearing: never having a child or having the first born after the age of 30

- obesity: the body is able to convert body fat and testosterone (higher in obese women) to estrogen
- birth control pills: In the past, studies suggested a potential relationship between birth control pills and an increased risk for breast cancer. Doses of estrogen used in the 1960s were much higher than the doses used today. Long-time pill use, especially during the vulnerable years (before the first pregnancy), may increase the risk. More studies are needed to determine whether there is a relationship between current birth control pill use and breast cancer.
- HRT for postmenopausal women: Many observational studies have suggested that use of hormone replacement therapy for more than 5 years is associated with an increased risk for hormone-related breast cancers.

**Diet and nutrition.** What you eat appears to play a role in breast cancer risk. Many researchers question the relationship between high-fat diets and breast cancer by studying women in different countries. For example, women in Japan who eat a lower-fat diet have lower rates of breast cancer than do women in the United States. As women from other countries with low rates of breast cancer become more westernized (eat our foods), the rate of breast cancer increases. The daughters of these women have even higher rates of breast cancer, which suggests that exposure during the younger, more vulnerable years is a major risk factor.

Other studies in adult women have found a weak or no relationship between high-fat foods and breast cancer. Some experts believe that the type of fat may make a difference. Others suggest that the increase in risk is related to weight gain, which leads to obesity. There are no conclusive studies showing the relationship between fat consumption and risk, but eating lots of vegetables may help protect you against cancer.

**Drinking.** Drinking 2 or more alcoholic drinks a day may increase your risk of breast cancer. There are a number of studies supporting the claim that alcohol increases a woman's risk. Alcohol can be converted into estrogen. The results from the Nurse's Health Study suggest that women who consumed 3–9 alcoholic drinks a week had a 30% increased risk of breast cancer and those who had more than 9 drinks a week had a 60% increased risk. The greatest risk was in thin women. Findings from a few other studies suggest that there may be more of a risk for women who consume large amounts of alcohol during the younger, more vulnerable years.

## Do women with diabetes have a greater risk for developing breast cancer?

We don't know. It appears that women with diabetes may have endocrine factors that can influence the growth of hormone-related breast tumors. One study, published in 1998, did report that post-menopausal women with a family history of diabetes had more risk factors for breast cancer *but did not have more breast cancer*. This population based study looked at more than 41,000 women with and without diabetes between the ages of 55–69 years of age for 10 years. Researchers did not find a relation between having a family history of diabetes and a family history of breast cancer. The findings of the study did show that there might be more breast cancer in women with diabetes who have a sister with breast cancer.

None of the studies are conclusive. Until the relationship of diabetes to breast cancer is better understood, women are advised to reduce the risk factors that are known to increase their risk and to have routine breast exams.

## What can I do to prevent breast cancer?

Recommendations for preventing breast cancer include yearly screening for early detection and treatment, regular exercise, and healthy eating.

## Screening for breast cancer

Early detection and treatment of breast cancer is critical. This means doing breast self exams (BSE), having routine breast exams from a health care professional, and having routine mammograms.

**Breast self exams (BSE).** Breast self exams are a most critical health habit to adopt. Doing an exam every month means looking at and feeling for changes in your breasts. This allows you to get to know your breasts, so that if something changes, you will know it. The best time to do a self-exam is 7–10 days after the first day of your period. It may be necessary to have your health care provider show you how to do this exam. If you are unsure whether you are doing it correctly, please ask for help.

**Professional breast exams.** It is important to have a physical exam that includes an exam of your breasts. This involves looking and feeling for changes. It you believe that there is a problem with a breast, be sure to point it out to your doctor.

**Mammograms.** Mammograms usually are more accurate in detecting a breast lump in women older than 50. This is because the breast tissue is fattier and less dense then. The more dense the breast, the more difficult it is to interpret the results of the mammogram. Before the exam don't use any powders, deodorants, or creams on your breasts or on your underarms. They tend to interfere with the clarity of the test. The chart below outlines the

| Exam | 50 years and older | 40–50 years | 20–39 |
|---|---|---|---|
| BSE | Every month | Every month | Every month |
| Professional Breast Exam | Every year | Every 1–2 years depending on risk | Every 1–3 years depending on risk |
| Mammogram | Every year | Every 2 years depending on risk | |

recommendations for breast exams from the American Cancer Society, American College of Obstetricians, and American Medical Association. If you have had a sister or mother with breast cancer, you will want to be screened more frequently and earlier.

### Exercise and nutrition

Observational studies have shown that women who exercise regularly may have a lower risk of breast cancer. Remember, because this is a population-based study, there is a possibility that the women who exercise are more health conscious and eat healthier, too. More exercise may also help a woman to be leaner and reduce the effects of being overweight. In general, it is recommended that a woman consume a low-fat, high-fiber meal plan, consume lots of vegetables and fruits, and limit alcohol to 3–5 drinks a week. In addition she may want to supplement her diet with antioxidants, such as vitamins A, C, and E. The meal plan that you are already following for diabetes control should help you reduce your risk of developing breast cancer.

## Osteoporosis and Healthy Bones

We have all seen women (and some men) who, as they aged, developed a dowager's hump, a hump in the back that causes them to stoop forward. Many women also mistakenly believe that it is normal and expected to lose height with age. Experts in the field of bone disease have come to appreciate that the dowager's hump and height loss do not necessarily have to happen. Thanks to studies on various medications, researchers and experts are learning more about how to prevent and treat the condition we know as osteoporosis.

### What is osteoporosis and why is it important to you?

Osteoporosis means porous bone. As we age, especially after we start losing estrogen, our bone mass decreases and the quality of our bone can become poor. This can lead to fragile bones and, if left untreated, may result in wrist, spinal, and hip fractures. A woman with fragile bones can suffer a spinal fracture just by coughing or reaching down to pick up a bag of groceries or her grandchild. This occurs because the quality of the bone in the vertebrae is weak and collapses. Multiple spine fractures can lead to the hump that we spoke of earlier. Living with spinal fracture can be difficult and painful. Hip fractures are more likely to occur in our 70s and 80s and can alter a woman's independence and quality of life. So it is important to prevent osteoporosis.

Our bones are the structure that holds our body together, supported by muscles and ligaments. If we do not maintain the quality of that bone, it will begin to get thin and weak. Compare bone to the struts and braces used to build a home. To withstand pressure, builders use thick struts. This is like the density of your bone. They also use material that won't break down easily. This is like the quality of your bone.

Initially the wrist and spine are more susceptible for fracture because they are made primarily of bone that looks like latticework that has a thin hard shell around it. The hip is made of bone that is solid and dense. Bone is alive and dynamic. It is always undergoing a change to keep healthy. Old bone is removed while new bone is laid down and replaced at a constant rate. As we age, the rate of new bone growth decreases dramatically, but the removal of old bone continues. If a woman doesn't take steps to reduce the rate of removal, the bone mass becomes thinner and weaker. The structure of the bone becomes poor. This leads to fragile bones, looking similar to the old, fine lace on your grandmother's bureaus. The good news is that we know how to slow down the removal process.

## How can I know whether I have osteoporosis?

For the most part, osteoporosis has no early symptoms. It is considered a silent disease. It doesn't happen overnight, and not everyone gets it. It develops over decades, starting in our 40s–50s, the period of time that we begin to lose estrogen. Peak bone mass is usually attained somewhere in our mid 30s. During the 5–6 years after menopause, a woman can lose bone mass rapidly as a result of estrogen deficiency—if she doesn't take the necessary steps to preserve her bone! The rate of bone loss slows down after that.

How quickly (and whether) you develop osteoporosis is influenced by many factors, including how much bone mass you acquired in early adulthood. If you enter the menopausal years with high bone mass (or high bone density), you will be less likely to develop osteoporosis than a woman who enters the menopausal years with low bone mass.

To help you determine whether you have or are at risk for developing osteoporosis, you may need to have a bone scan to measure your bone density. The bone density test called the DXA Scan (Dual Energy X-Ray Absorptiometry) usually scans either the spine or the hip. The test is not painful and is usually covered by health insurance. It involves you lying quietly on a table as a machine scans your spine or hip. The DXA scan gives a score that is used to compare the density of your bone to that of a young, healthy woman (peak bone mass). This score is referred to as the "t-score." The lower the bone mass, the lower the t-score and the higher the risk for fracture. It is generally recommended that you have bone scan done during the menopausal years.

There are different techniques to measure the density or quality of your bone, and they will provide different results. The different sites that are measured also provide different results. For example, a t-score of −2.5 of the spine does not equal a t-score of −2.5 of the hip. In addition, bone loss occurs at different rates at different sites. You may be classified as having osteoporosis in one site and

---

### T-scores of a bone density test of the spine using DXA

Normal is a score over −1.0
Osteopenia (low bone mass) is a score between −2.5 and −1.0.
(If ignored, it can progress to osteoporosis.)
Osteoporosis is a score of −2.5 or lower.

normal in another. That is why it is very important to work with physicians and technicians who are specially trained in determining what site is best to measure as well as how to interpret what the score means for you. After 65 years of age, spine density may naturally increase as a result of age. That's why most physicians will choose to measure the hip for bone density.

Some experts feel that an ultrasound of the heel or forearm may be helpful as a screening tool. Yet, to provide you with a more accurate diagnosis of osteoporosis, a DXA scan of the spine or hip is needed. If you receive a score of −1.0 or lower using an ultrasound device, you will more than likely need a DXA scan to get a better idea of your fracture risk.

Experts in the field of osteoporosis are working to improve the guidelines for interpreting the results from different devices, techniques, and sites. Until that is done, it is advised that you seek the expertise of a bone expert for this interpretation.

## Who is at risk?

**Genetics.** If you have a grandmother, mother, or sister with osteoporosis or a fracture that was not the cause of a major trauma, you are at risk as well. The diagnosis may never have been made, but you might be suspicious if you remember any of them having lost a lot of height as they aged or if they had the dowager's hump.

**Age.** As we age our risk increases. Postmenopausal women are at increased risk because their production of estrogen is dramatically reduced.

**Body types.** Women who have bigger muscles and heavier bones have a lower risk. Bigger muscles put more stress on the bones, forcing the bone to be stronger. Thinner women are more at risk than heavier women. Heavier women are more protected from osteoporosis. The body can convert substances in fat cells into estrogen. This helps to preserve the bone mass.

**Race.** African Americans and Mexican Americans tend to have thicker bones when they enter the menopausal years. As a result, even though they will lose bone after menopause, they will have started at a higher level, and it will take longer for them to reach the levels that are at risk for fractures. This does not mean that they are not at risk for osteoporosis. It just means that they are more likely to develop osteoporosis later than Caucasian and Asian women.

**Medications.** Steroids interfere with the development of new bone. They prevent calcium from being absorbed and increases the amount of calcium lost in the urine. Long-term steroid use requires supplementation with calcium and vitamin D. Treatment with osteoporosis drugs may also be necessary.

Other medications that you might take too much of such as thyroid medication, anti-seizure medications, diuretics, and antacids can promote bone loss or interfere with bone rebuilding. Use of sedative drugs may impair your coordination and increase your risk for falls.

**Nutrition.** Calcium and vitamin D are critical for healthy bones. Vitamin D and parathyroid hormones help to keep the levels of calcium in balance. Your ability to absorb calcium decreases with age. Most women take in only one-third to one-half of the amount of calcium needed on a daily basis, making calcium supplementation necessary.

Without vitamin D, the body cannot use calcium effectively. Vitamin D helps the absorption of calcium from the intestines. It also helps the kidneys to reabsorb the calcium into the blood stream. Vitamin D is best obtained from the sun. But when people use sun-blocking agents, the skin is less exposed to the sun and unable to make enough vitamin D. Women who live in northern climates or who stay indoors a great deal of the time tend to have lower vitamin D levels, too. This is especially true during the winter months. Daily supplementation of 400–800 IUs of vitamin D may be necessary. Check with your health care provider.

Heavy alcohol use may interfere with coordination and balance and can increase a woman's risk for falls and injury. Women who consume large amounts of alcohol may also not take in enough of the nutrients they need.

**Lifestyle.** Smoking cigarettes is toxic to the bone. Smoking stimulates the breakdown of estrogen, making estrogen less available and effective. It also interferes with the beneficial effects of hormone replacement therapy.

Weight-bearing types of exercise stress the bone and force muscle to contract. This in turn stimulates more bone to form. Lack of any exercise, especially of the weight- bearing type, increases a woman's risk for low bone mass.

**Medical conditions or health states.** Women with shorter exposure to their own estrogen are at increased risk for osteoporosis. Women who go through menopause early (30s and 40s) are at risk because they have been without their own estrogen for a longer period of time. Having had a total hysterectomy (surgical menopause) puts women at risk because their source of estrogen, the ovaries, have been suddenly removed. Women who go through natural menopause lose their estrogen slowly, so they benefit from its protective effects for a little longer. Women with menstrual irregularity and fewer pregnancies are also at increased risk.

There are conditions that interfere with the absorption of nutrients that build bone. Women with eating disorders such as anorexia or bulimia may not receive the nutrients to make their own estrogen, putting them at risk for losing bone much earlier than women without eating disorders. Other conditions include having had stomach surgery, certain types of cancer or cancer treatment, hyperactive thyroid or too much thyroid medication, Cushing Syndrome, and type 1 diabetes.

**Diabetes.** Women with type 2 diabetes are thought to be less at risk for developing osteoporosis because most women with type 2 diabetes are overweight. Some studies have shown that women with type 2 diabetes have higher bone densities. Other studies show otherwise. The differences noted in these studies may be related to whether the women studied were heavy or thin and whether they had had diabetes for a short time or a longer period of time. More studies with larger numbers of women with type 2 diabetes are needed to determine whether they have an increased risk or a normal risk for osteoporosis. The role of blood sugar control and the risk for bone loss is not well understood. There are several studies that suggest high concentrations of blood sugar in women with type 2 diabetes interfere with the cells that help to build new bone. Other studies suggest that there is no relationship.

A number of studies have shown that women with type 1 diabetes tend to have lower bone mass and more osteoporosis than women without diabetes. It is believed that low bone mass is related, in part, to the lack of insulin early on in the development of diabetes. People with type 1 diabetes no longer produce their own insulin. Insulin is needed for calcium to be absorbed. As the levels of insulin become lower, the body is unable to absorb calcium effectively, which leads to low bone mass. In addition, many women with type 1 diabetes are thin and Caucasian, which we know to be strong risk factors for osteoporosis.

The specific causes of low bone density in women with type 1 diabetes are unknown. It is unclear whether there is a role between blood sugar control, duration of diabetes, and coexisting complications, and the risk for low bone density. Some researchers speculate that women with type 1 diabetes may not achieve peak bone mass the way women without diabetes do. Others feel that the diabetic woman may lose bone mass more rapidly after peak bone mass is attained. More studies are needed to help answer these questions.

There are two conditions known to cause osteoporosis, hyperparathyroidism and hyperthyroidism (Grave's disease). These conditions are more common in women with diabetes. Because of this, it is important for a woman to have routine blood tests to check her thyroid function and to receive proper treatment if abnormal. The presence of these conditions may explain why some women with diabetes suffer more bone loss.

**Risk for fractures.** Problems that do not increase your risk for osteoporosis but increase your risk for fractures are neuropathy (damage to the nerves) and loss of vision. Women with osteoporosis or low bone mass who also have neuropathy may be at risk for falling and suffering a fracture. As the nerves become damaged, they are unable to stimulate the muscles to stay firm, leading to changes in the shape of your feet and problems with walking. Not being able to see where you are walking or problems with depth perception may increase your chances for falls and subsequent fractures.

Over the last few years, studies have shown that women who have an existing fracture are at risk for having another. If you have had a fracture after the age of 50 years that was unrelated to major trauma, your risk for another one is very high. Taking medication and adopting health practices to prevent another fracture is critical.

## *Combination of risks*

The more risk factors you have, the greater the chance of developing osteoporosis and fractures. If you have type 1 diabetes, have an eating disorder, or have very high $HbA_{1c}$ levels, your risk for losing bone mass and developing osteoporosis increases.

| Risk Factors |
| --- |
| Family history |
| Caucasian, Northern European, Asian |
| Small, thin frame |
| Postmenopausal, early or surgical menopause |
| Physical inactivity |
| Smoker |
| Diet low in calcium and vitamin D |
| Conditions interfering with nutrient absorption |
| Medications interfering with bone strength and quality |
| Type 1 diabetes |

## *What can I do to prevent or treat osteoporosis?*

Before menopause, try the ways to increase bone mass and maximize your bone density (such as healthy eating and regular weight-bearing exercise) before you lose the protective effects of estrogen. During and after menopause, continue eating well and weight-bearing exercise and look into treatments that counteract the effects of loss of estrogen. If you have low bone mass (osteopenia) or osteoporosis, you and your doctor may want to consider medications that can help prevent further bone loss.

Make sure that you have adequate calcium and vitamin D in your diet. If you are premenopausal or are taking estrogen, ensure that you are getting 1,000–1,300 mg/day of calcium and 400–800 IU of vitamin D a day. If you are postmenopausal and not taking HRT, calcium intake should be 1,500 mg a day. Some research suggests that magnesium also helps you absorb calcium, about 400 mg/day if you are getting the recommended amount of calcium. If you are unable to get the recommended amounts of these nutrients through food, use supplements. See hints on taking calcium.

Engage in weight-bearing exercises to strengthen muscles such as lifting small weights (½ to 1 pound to begin). Don't worry, you won't get big bulging muscles from weight lifting. What you will get is

---

### Hints On Taking Calcium

For maximizing absorption and reducing side effects, do not take your calcium all at once and do take it with food. Take half in the morning and half in the afternoon or evening. If you are having trouble with constipation or bloating, even after splitting the dose, consider changing to a preparation that has calcium citrate. You might try crushing it and taking it in orange juice. It is preferable to take a calcium supplement that is easily absorbed and has the highest available calcium per tablet. Calcium carbonate is the preferred source of calcium because it has the highest calcium per tablet.

---

smooth, toned muscle, which is heavier than fat and helps you hold on to more bone. Walking, especially brisk walking, is a weight-bearing exercise! Other examples are jogging, tennis, in-line skating, and skiing. Swimming and bicycle riding are not considered weight bearing, but they are excellent aerobic exercises to round out your efforts. More and more studies are showing that leading an active lifestyle helps to reduce the risk for spinal and hip fractures.

In *The Osteoporosis Book* Nancy Lane reports that women who have not exercised can increase their bone density by 3–4% by starting an exercise program that includes lifting hand weights and walking briskly for 30 minutes, 3–4 times a week. Some women try to combine these activities and carry the weights or wear them around their ankles while they are walking, but that isn't a good idea. It puts unusual strain on the joints at the shoulder, elbow, wrist, ankle, and knee. If you want to carry more weight for the bone-building benefit, put them in a backpack.

It is also important to engage in activities such as yoga or tai-chi that increase your flexibility, strength, and balance. They multiply the benefits of your other types of exercise to make you stronger and healthier. Flexibility exercises also help decrease your risk for falls and injury.

Work on reducing your risk by stopping smoking and reducing your intake of alcohol. If you have an eating disorder, seek the help of professionals who can support your efforts in healing.

Know how to reduce your risk for falling, especially if you have neuropathy or visual loss. If you have problems with balance, walking, muscle weakness of your legs or neuropathy, talk to your health care providers to learn about devices you might use to provide more stability. Consider asking for a consult with a physical therapist who can teach you exercises to strengthen your muscles and reduce your risks for falls. To test your strength and coordination, try rising from a chair 5 or more times without using the arms. If you are unable to do this, you might benefit from strengthening exercises. The nice thing is that even in our 90s, we can begin lifting 1-pound weights and doing strengthening exercises and increase our muscle mass just as younger people do. It's literally never too late.

If you have visual problems that put you at risk, work with your health care team to find out about the resources available to help you. Look at ways to eliminate clutter or unnecessary items in your home or work place that might increase the risk of tripping or falling.

## *Medications*

Most experts believe that if you are at increased risk for osteoporosis and your bone density score is low, calcium and vitamin D alone cannot protect you from fractures. Combining calcium and vitamin D with a medication that either builds bone or reduces the rate that it is broken down is usually recommended. Keep in mind that if you stop the medication, the positive effects will be lost soon after it is discontinued. None of the studies to date have included large numbers of women with type 1 or type 2 diabetes. So experts

---

### Drugs that Build or Save Bone

**Calcitonin (miacalcin)**

In one study that looked at women who were 15–22 years post menopause, 200 mg of Calcitonin a day was shown to decrease their risk for fractures by 40%. Calcitonin decreases the rate that bone is broken down. There is still some debate about the true effectiveness of this drug. Studies are under way to help answer some unresolved questions.
- It is delivered as a nasal spray.
- Major side effect is nausea and mild gastrointestinal discomfort.
- It has also been shown to alleviate bone pain.

**Evista (raloxifene)**

Evista has been shown to increase bone density. In the MORE trial (Multiple Outcomes for Raloxifene Evaluation) more than 7,700 women with osteoporosis were randomized to receive Evista or a placebo for 4 years. The results of this study showed that Evista helped to reduce the risk for fracture by 55% in women who did not have a previous spinal fracture and 30% in women who did have a previous fracture.

---

- Evista can be taken easily at any time of day, with or without food.
- Evista also has been shown to lower LDL and total cholesterol and reduce the risk of estrogen-positive breast cancer in women with osteoporosis. It does not cause stimulation of the uterine wall or increase the risk for uterine cancer.
- Major side effects include an increased risk for mild-moderate hot flashes and deep vein blood clots. Hot flashes were more likely to occur in women who were recently menopausal or had a history of hot flashes. The occurrence of deep vein blood clots was rare and similar to that seen in women treated with HRT.

### Fosamax (alendronate)
In two randomized clinical trials, referred to as the FIT trials (Fracture Intervention Trial), Fosamax was shown to reduce the risk for fracture by about 50% in women who did not have a previous fracture and 90% in women with a previous fracture. In one of the trials, Fosamax reduced the risk for hip fractures in women who were older and who had a previous spinal fracture.
- Fosamax must be taken in the morning on an empty stomach. Once taken with water, a woman must remain upright for at least 30 minutes.
- Fosamax only works on the bone. It does not affect the heart, breast, or uterus.
- Major side effects include increased risk for upper gastric irritation like heartburn or pain and esophagitis.

### Hormone Replacement Therapy
There have been several observational studies suggesting that estrogen and the combination of estrogen and progestin are effective in decreasing the risk for spinal and hip fractures. Many clinical trials have shown that both are effective in increasing bone density. There have been no randomized clinical trials done comparing hormone replacement therapy to placebo. For an in-depth discussion of hormone replacement therapy, see pages 158–169.

can only assume the benefits or risks are similar to women without diabetes.

The medications currently approved for the prevention of osteoporosis are Evista, Fosamax, and HRT. The medications currently approved for the treatment of osteoporosis are Calcitonin, Evista, Fosamax, and HRT.

## Matters of the Heart

Contrary to popular belief, heart disease is the leading cause of death and disability in women. One of three women will die of heart disease as compared to one of nine women dying of breast cancer. Forty percent of heart attacks result in death. Women who have heart attacks or undergo heart surgery tend not to do as well as men.

For decades people have believed that women are not at risk for developing heart disease until they have gone through menopause. This is not necessarily true, especially for women with diabetes. It is believed that estrogen provides a certain degree of protection against heart disease. Estrogen released from the ovaries helps to increase the production of HDL cholesterol (the good cholesterol) and to break down LDL cholesterol (the bad cholesterol). It also relaxes the smooth muscle of the blood vessels. Once a women experiences menopause, the production of estrogen goes down.

### Heart disease and diabetes

Diabetes is a powerful risk factor for heart disease in women. In the Nurse's Health Study, the researchers showed that women with diabetes were 3 to 7 times more likely to have heart disease and related problems. Heart disease is the leading cause of death in women with diabetes. As a woman with diabetes, you are at risk for developing heart disease earlier than your friends who don't have diabetes. The presence of diabetes negates or overrides the protective effect of estrogen, which results in heart disease being more common in women with diabetes, and it occurs when they are younger. Women with diabetes are twice as likely to have a second heart attack and 4 times more likely to have heart failure than women without diabetes.

Researchers are not clear why women with diabetes have more heart disease. But because you have diabetes, you are more likely to have abnormal blood fat levels, problems with clotting, and high blood pressure than are your friends who don't have diabetes. Any risk factor is more dangerous for a woman with diabetes. If you have high blood pressure (greater than 130/85), your chance of having heart problems is much greater than that of your friend who only has high blood pressure. Your risk for heart disease increases further if you have protein in your urine and currently smoke. High blood pressure and smoking is a very dangerous combination for a woman with diabetes! Elevated triglycerides appears to carry even more of a risk for the woman with diabetes.

Many women with type 2 diabetes already have heart disease when they are diagnosed or have many of the risk factors such as high lipid (blood fat) levels, high blood pressure, abdominal obesity, and abnormalities in blood vessel function. Women with type 1 diabetes can develop heart disease when they are young women. They tend to benefit less from their own body's estrogen. Being overweight or gaining weight can lead to abnormal blood fats. In a small study that looked at overweight women with type 1 diabetes, researchers found that women who improved blood sugar control had better blood fat levels. Those that did not improve control had unfavorable blood fat levels. These findings suggest that a woman's efforts in improving blood sugars by following a balanced meal plan or exercising pay off for her heart, too. Some studies also suggest that elevated $HbA_{1c}$ levels carry some increased risk.

## Symptoms

Heart attacks occur when the heart muscle doesn't get enough oxygen. This can be a life-threatening event, especially for a woman with diabetes. Knowing the symptoms of a heart attack is important. However, people with diabetes may not always feel these symptoms. Diabetes can damage the nerves that would normally give you the warning feelings of a serious heart problem. So, it is very important that you do not ignore any suspicious feelings! It is better to be seen by your doctor and find out that it is nothing than to let it go.

Signs and symptoms of heart disease can be misinterpreted or misdiagnosed. Women may present with symptoms different from men. Fatigue, indigestion, nausea (feeling sick to your stomach) and vomiting often can be the initial symptoms.

Sudden death may be more common in women than in men. There are many suggested reasons for this difference. Many women do not think that they are at risk. Others have vague symptoms that do not resemble what they consider the classical symptoms. Symptoms can come and go and easily be confused with other illnesses. Some women attempt to self-treat or just deny that something is wrong. Many women question themselves about their symptoms, particularly if they are not taken seriously by health care workers or their family. For all these reasons, many women delay seeking treatment.

To recognize the signs and symptoms of heart disease you need to know what they are. You need to believe in yourself, trusting and knowing that something is wrong and that you are worth having it checked out. Many women fear the condescending comments of others such as "See, I told you it was nothing." Such comments bring up confusion and distrust in our ability to trust ourselves. Keep trusting yourself.

A list of the symptoms of heart attack is given in the box on page 200. Symptoms common to women are marked with an asterisk. Your symptoms of a heart attack may be very different from a man's and may be misinterpreted as something else. Remember that because you have diabetes, you may not experience severe pain or pressure. The symptoms tend to be subtle. In the second box is a list of additional symptoms and signs that a woman with diabetes might experience. If you are concerned that you may be experiencing a heart attack, be persistent and make your needs known. You should expect, at a minimum, a physical exam, blood work, and an electrocardiogram (ECG).

### Knowing what puts you at risk

Doing what you can to prevent heart disease is the first step. We realize that this is not always possible. You may already have heart disease before you are diagnosed with diabetes. Even if you have heart disease, this section will help you try and prevent it from getting worse.

Smoking, being overweight or sedentary, having high blood pressure, or high cholesterol and triglycerides levels are major risk factors for heart disease. You can modify these to reduce your risk. You cannot do anything to change other factors such as family history and diabetes.

**Early family history of heart disease.** Having a father with heart disease before age 50 or a mother or sister before age 65 is a major risk factor.

**Smoking.** Smoking triples the risk for heart attack in women. Unfortunately, efforts to promote smoking cessation in women have not been very effective. Smoking increases the chances of your having a heart attack at a younger age and for going through menopause two years earlier. It lowers HDL levels. In the Nurses' Health Study, women who smoked more had poorer health than women who smoked less. When a woman stops smoking, she will decrease her risk of dying from heart disease by 24% in 2 years. Within 3–5 years, her risk will come closer to that of women who never smoke.

**High blood pressure.** It is estimated that 50% of Caucasian Americans and 80% of African Americans have high blood pressure. Controlling high blood pressure decreases the risk of stroke, heart attacks, and death. According to the ADA, the goal for blood pressure for most people with diabetes is less than 130/85. The goal for your blood pressure may be different if you have other health problems, such as kidney disease.

**Lipid abnormalities.** Low HDL levels can predict heart disease in women. For most women, HDL levels are higher than in men until well after menopause. The Framingham Heart Study, a population-based study, suggested that for every 10 mg/dl fall in HDL level, there was a 40–50% increase in risk for heart disease. So far, there has been no clinical trial to show that increasing HDL decreases risk. There are different types of HDL. $HDL_2$ and $HDL_3$ are believed to have different levels of cardio-protection.

LDL cholesterol also increases after menopause and is found to be a predictor of death and disease. LDL size and density is also important. Statin drugs such as Mevacor, Lipitor, Zocor, Pravacol, and Lescol are often prescribed for treatment of high lipid levels. Studies have shown that a reduction in LDL was beneficial for both men and women. See page 201 for a description of these studies.

Some studies have suggested that elevated triglycerides are an independent risk factor for women, more so than for men. Other studies are not as convincing. What the studies do show is that the combination of low HDL levels and high tryiglycerides are problematic for all women.

The relationship between HDL, LDL, and triglycerides is more complex that first meets the eye. More research is being done to find out what types and what levels of blood fats are important in the prevention of heart disease.

**Homocysteine.** Homocysteine is an amino acid produced during metabolism of food. Population-based studies suggested that elevated levels of homocysteine are linked with an increased risk for heart disease. Currently it is thought that high levels of homocysteine are linked to the formation of oxygen-free radicals that can cause damage to the blood vessels. Homocysteine levels can be reduced by taking B-vitamins (such as a pill containing folic acid, vitamin B-6, and vitamin-B12). So far, there has not been a study to show that reducing homocysteine levels will result in a reduction in risk for heart disease.

**C-Reactive Protein.** People with unstable angina (chest pain) have higher levels of a protein that is associated with inflammation and are more likely to have a heart attack than people with lower levels. This protein is called C-Reactive protein. In some studies, an elevation in C-Reactive protein may increase the risk of heart attack as much as seven times. More studies are needed to determine how this protein is involved with heart disease.

**Central obesity: waist-to-hip ratio.** The waist-to-hip ratio refers to the difference in the measurements of your hip and waist. If they are nearly the same size or your waist is bigger than your hips, you have a high waist-to-hip ratio. A high waist-to-hip ratio means that you have more abdominal body fat, and your body shape is more like an apple. Having an apple shaped body is associated with heart disease.

**Lifestyle.** Some experts have seen an increased risk in women who perceive their lifestyle or job as stressful. Studies looking at the impact of activity on cardiac risk have found that women— young and old—who participated in physical activity reduced their risk for heart disease by 50%. What is most exciting about the new research is that exercising for 10 minutes 3 times a day, 5–6 days a week may be as effective in reducing risk as exercising for 30–45 minutes 3–4 times a week.

**Other health problems.** It appears that women who have a history of polycystic ovary syndrome (PCOS) tend to have heart disease. Women with PCOS, have higher levels of testosterone and other male hormones. They also have higher waist-to-hip ratios and insulin resistance, all of which are believed to put a woman at increased risk.

**Depression.** Recent studies have suggested that there might be a correlation between depression and heart disease in women. It is unclear why this is. One possibility is that depression leads to decreased attention to self-care, feeling hopeless, and not following the treatment plan. Chinese medicine suggests that the emotional "aching" heart translates physically as a real aching heart.

Whatever the relationship is, it is important for women to pay attention to the presence of depression and seek out appropriate treatment.

## *Know your numbers*

Get specific information about your own risk profile. Once you know your risks, you can learn to reduce them and prevent further problems. You will need to know your lipid levels, blood pressure, and cardiac-risk ratio. Use the grid on page 199 to keep track of your risk profile.

A cardiac-risk ratio is a way of determining how likely you are to have a heart attack soon. Ask your doctor to help you calculate and interpret your own cardiac-risk ratio. Use the equation below. A number of 3.5 or below means that your risk is low. A score of 6 or higher means that your risk is very high and you should see your health care provider soon!

$$\text{cardiac risk ratio} = \frac{\text{cholesterol level}}{\text{HDL level}}$$

Example: If cholesterol is 210 mg/dl and HDL is 50,

$$\text{cardiac risk ratio} = \frac{210}{50} = 4.2$$

See the box on the page 200 for a description of the risk factors common to many women with diabetes. Keep in mind that having these risk factors does not make you feel different or badly. That is why routine screening by your health care provider is important.

## *Taking action*

Start reducing your individual risk today! To have the greatest impact, it is important for a woman with diabetes to stop smoking and to get her blood pressure under control. Healthy life practices such as yoga and meditation combined with a healthy lifestyle of physical activity and good nutrition are sure ways of strengthening your heart and blood vessels. Fiber is important in reducing cholesterol and triglycerides. Exercise increases muscle, which in turn reduces the blood fat and blood sugar levels. More muscle means more calories burned, even when you're resting!

## Beta-blockers

Studies also show that if you have had a heart attack, your risk for another heart attack or death may be reduced if you take a beta-blocker, such as Lopressor or Carvedilol. But if you are taking medication, you should continue treatments proven to reduce cardiac risk, such as lowering blood pressure and cholesterol and exercising regularly.

## Aspirin

Most experts believe that low-dose aspirin therapy is beneficial in preventing the first heart attack in diabetes patients who are at high risk and for reducing the risk for a second heart attack in diabetes patients who have already had a heart attack. Because women with diabetes are at high risk for developing heart disease, they are often advised to take one low-dose aspirin a day, as long as no contraindications exist.

Aspirin use does have some risk, such as gastric irritation and bleeding, and in some cases, stroke. Aspirin is not advised for women who have aspirin allergies, bleeding tendencies, who are on anticoagulant therapy like Coumadin, who have had GI bleeding, or have active liver disease.

The ADA has endorsed the use of a low-dose (85–325 mg) aspirin a day for women who have large vessel disease, such as a history of a heart attack, by-pass surgery, stroke or TIAs (small strokes), poor circulation, claudication, or angina.

In addition, they recommend considering aspirin therapy for women who

- have a family history of heart disease
- are cigarette smokers
- have high blood pressure

- are obese
- have protein in the urine
- have cholesterol levels over 200, LDL levels over 130, HDL levels lower than 40, and triglycerides over 250

It is very important to seek medical evaluation at the first sign of angina (chest pain), difficult breathing, sweating, or nausea. Delay in seeking care may complicate your recovery.

## *Hormone replacement therapy*

The effect of HRT on heart disease is still not determined. Some studies have found that progestins may cause insulin resistance, leading to higher blood sugars. Adjustments in diabetes medications can be made to accommodate this if it happens. Recently, there were a few studies looking at the effect of estrogen taken for 6–12 weeks in postmenopausal women with diabetes. Blood sugar levels and $HbA_{1c}$ levels were lower, and blood fats improved as well. In two studies the triglyceride levels did not go up. In one study they did. It is important to remember that these results may not apply to post-menopausal women treated with combination hormone therapy.

As a woman with diabetes you need to take your risk for heart disease seriously. Aggressive treatment of risk factors and prompt treatment for symptoms is critical for your health.

---

### Risk Factors for Heart Disease for the General Public

Family history of heart disease
Smoking
High blood pressure: greater than 130/85 mmHg
High triglycerides: greater than 200 mg/dl
LDL cholesterol: greater than 130 mg/dl
HDL cholesterol: less than 35 mg/dl
Cardiac-risk ratio: greater than 3.5 for women
Sedentary lifestyle
Overweight (greater than 120% over desired weight)

---

| Classic Symptoms of Heart Attack |
|---|
| • Shortness of breath<br>• Pain or tightness in your chest wall, jaw, or back of neck or down the right or left arm<br>• Aching, throbbing, or a squeezing sensation*<br>• Weakness, fatigue or drowsiness*<br>• Hot poker tab in the chest*<br>• Feeling like the heart jumps into the throat*<br>• Heartbeat feeling like it is racing or skipping*<br>• Nausea |
| **Additional Symptoms** |
| • Blood sugar values suddenly out of control<br>• Vomiting<br>• Confusion<br>• Extreme fatigue<br>*common to women |

| Common Risk Profile for Women<br>with Type 2 Diabetes |
|---|
| Diabetes<br>High blood pressure: greater than 130/85<br>Abnormal blood fats:<br>    Low HDL, less than 40 mg/dl<br>    High triglycerides<br>    High cholesterol<br>Weight gain around the waist: having an apple-shaped body<br>    instead of a pear-shaped body<br>Sedentary lifestyle |
| **Common Risk Profile for Women<br>with Type 1 Diabetes** |
| Diabetes |

# Heart Studies

Over the last several years, there have been studies looking at the effect of estrogen and lipid-lowering drugs in reducing the risk for heart disease and heart attacks in women. Changes in blood vessel walls, the inability to dilate, and increase in blood clotting factors are highly predictive of heart disease. Studies of estrogen use in women show that estrogen helps to improve ability of the blood vessel wall to dilate and decrease the likelihood of clots sticking to the vessel wall. It is not known whether or not estrogen can improve these conditions in women with diabetes. These studies are under way.

Researchers have studied the effects of drugs called ACE-inhibitors. One such study called the HOPE study (Heart Outcomes Prevention Evaluation) found these drugs to be very effective in reducing death related to heart disease, heart attack, stroke, and the need for procedures like angioplasties in women with vascular disease and diabetes. It appears that these drugs help to improve blood pressure and prevent the formation of plaque ruptures.

Statins are lipid-lowering drugs currently available for the treatment of "dyslipidemia" or elevated cholesterol and triglycerides. Until recently, there were limited data available on women. There are 4 studies that looked at the effects of statins on the treatment and prevention of death related to heart disease. In 3 of the studies, women already had elevated cholesterol levels and heart disease. In the fourth study, they only had elevated cholesterol. The names of these studies are CARE (Cholesterol And Recurrent Events), LIPID study, AFCAPS (Air Force/Texas Coronary Atherosclerosis Prevention Study) and the 4S study (Scandinavian Simvastatin Survival Study). Results from these studies all show that women taking statins had a reduction in triglycerides, total cholesterol, and LDL levels, and an increase in HDL. This is good news for women, especially women with diabetes.

The National Cholesterol Education Program guidelines suggest that drug therapy be considered in postmenopausal women who have high LDL levels or multiple risk factors. Having diabetes is a major risk factor. The American Heart Association and American College of Cardiology recommend treatment of abnormal lipids with statin drugs.

Uncontrolled diabetes, high blood pressure, and high cholesterol put Tracy at risk for problems with circulation. She has had type 2 diabetes for many years.

*I take insulin twice a day. I am still 30 pounds overweight. I had two heart attacks and one stroke. After a lot of rehab, I am pretty independent. My husband is a great help. He is always asking me to go out for a walk. I am now retired, so my day is not as hectic.*

Tracy had many risk factors for heart disease. She did not appreciate how important it was to pay attention to her diabetes and blood pressure. This is common, especially when you don't feel bad. She did not realize how tired and sluggish she was. Today, she is working with her husband to improve her wellness.

Wellness is not defined by lack of illness or by physical health. It is an attitude. Tracy has a wonderful viewpoint on her current health.

*I still consider myself healthy. I am able to say that I have high blood pressure, high cholesterol, and diabetes. I believe that if I am able to do for myself and to get out of bed every morning, I am healthy. I thank God that I can enjoy my kids and grandkids.*

Tracy's attitude is healthy and honoring! She is no longer denying that she has diabetes. It is a part of her that needs to be cared for and nurtured. Small steps lead her forward to big changes.

*I know that I need to eat less, and I try. I wish I had made healthier food choices 5 and 10 years ago. Maybe I wouldn't have the problems I do today. But when things get tough, I pick myself up and start all over again.*

Change comes slowly. It isn't easy to change old behaviors. It is impossible to change what has happened in the past. Being realistic and less critical is an important step. No matter how small, each step takes you closer to your goal.

## Your Total Health Program

As a woman with diabetes you need to pay attention to your total health profile as well as to your diabetes. Ignoring one aspect of your health will compromise your ability to achieve wellness. In the following list, we have summarized the areas of physical health that are important for you to consider.

### Reproductive health
- If you are sexually active, use forms of contraception that prevent sexually transmitted disease (male or female condoms)
- Avoid multiple sex partners
- Plan your pregnancies
- Have a Pap smear every 1–3 years
- Participate in breast health practices
  - monthly breast self exams
  - professional breast exams
  - mammograms
- Stop smoking
- Limit alcohol intake

### Heart health
- Eat a low-fat (healthy fats) meal plan
- Engage in aerobic exercise regularly

- Live an active lifestyle
- Stop smoking
- Keep blood pressure under control, less than 130/85
- Control lipid levels: LDL < 130, HDL > 45, CHOL < 200, TRIG < 200
- Take medications as prescribed
- Maintain healthy weight

## Bone health

- 1,000–1,500 mg of calcium a day and 400–800 IU of vitamin D a day
- Engage in weight-bearing exercise routinely
- Get a bone density scan after menopause
- Take medications as prescribed
- Take measures to reduce the risk for falls
- Stop smoking
- Limit alcohol

## Colon health

- Eat a meal plan high in fiber and vegetables
- Get rectal exam and fecal stool samples done every 1–3 years
- If you are over age 50, ask your doctor about screening for colon cancer with a sigmoidoscopy or colonoscopy

## Diabetes health

- Keep $HbA_{1c}$ levels as close to normal as is possible
- Learn as much as you can about the ongoing changes in treatment options
- Eat a healthy meal plan
- Exercise regularly
- Check blood glucose levels at home
- If you take insulin, learn how to adjust your insulin on your own
- Treat high and low blood sugars promptly
- Have the following screening tests done yearly
  – dilated eye exam

- urine and blood tests to measure for kidney disease: micro-albuminuria and serum creatinine
- nerve sensation and function
- circulation
- blood pressure
• Take medications as prescribed

We hope that you give yourself the time and energy you deserve to be as healthy as you possibly can be. You are worth it!

# Resources

For more information about women's health issues, see the following books. They are excellent resources and provide you with detailed discussions about the health issues described in this chapter. You should be able to find them in a library or bookstore in the women's health or health improvement sections.

## Heart disease

*Woman and Heart Disease.* Edward B. Diethrich, MD, and Carol Cohan, Ballantine Books, New York, 1994.

*Women, Take Heart.* Richard H. Helfant, MD, G. P. Putnam's Sons, New York, 1993.

## Overall health

*New Passages: Mapping Your Life Across Time.* Gail Sheehy, Random House, New York, 1995.

*Women's Bodies, Women's Wisdom: Creating Physical and Emotional Health and Healing.* Christiane Northrup, MD, Bantam Books, New York, 1994.

*The New Our Bodies, Ourselves.* The Boston Women's Health Book Collective, Simon and Schuster, Inc., New York, 1984.

*The Diabetic Woman.* Lois Jovanovic, MD, June Biermann, Barbara Toohey, Jeremy P. Tarcher, Inc., Los Angeles, 1987.

## Breast health

Dr. Susan Love's Breast Book. Susan Love, MD, with Karen Lindsey, Addison-Wesley Publishing Co., St. Louis, 1995.

## Menopause

Menopause: All Your Questions Answered. Raymond G. Brunett, MD, Contemporary Books, Inc., Chicago, 1987.

Menopause, Naturally: Preparing for the Second Half of Life. Sadja Greenwood, MD, Volcano House, Volcano, California, 1992.

Menopausal Years: The Wise Woman Way. Susun S. Weed, Ash Tree Publishing, New York, 1992.

Passage to Power: Natural Menopause Revolution. Leslie Kenton, Hay House Inc., Carlsbad, California, 1995.

The Silent Passage. Gail Sheehy, Pocket Books, Simon and Schuster, Inc., New York, 1998.

## Hormone replacement therapy

Estrogen. Lila E. Nachtigall, MD, and Joan Rattner Heilman, Harper Perennial, New York, 1991.

The Estrogen Alternative. Steven R. Goldstein, MD, and Laurie Asner, G.P. Putnam's Sons, New York, 1998.

## Pregnancy

Diabetes and Pregnancy: What to Expect. American Diabetes Association, Alexandria, Virginia, 1996.

Gestational Diabetes: What to Expect. American Diabetes Association, Alexandria, Virginia, 1997.

## Osteoporosis

The Osteoporosis Book: A guide for patients and their families. Nancy E. Lane, MD, Oxford Univ. Press, New York, 1999.

## For questions about herbs

The American Association of Naturopathic Physicians (ND)
601 Valley, Suite 105
Seattle, WA 98109
(206) 298-0125
www.naturopathic.org

The American Herbalists Guild
6728 Old McLean Village Drive
McLean, VA 22101-3906
(703) 556-9728
www.holisticmedicine.org

The National Commission for Certification for Acupuncture and
   Oriental Medicine
11 Canal Center Plaza, Suite 300
Alexandria, VA 22314
(703) 548-9004
www.nccaom.org

# Chapter 7

# Life Practices that Matter

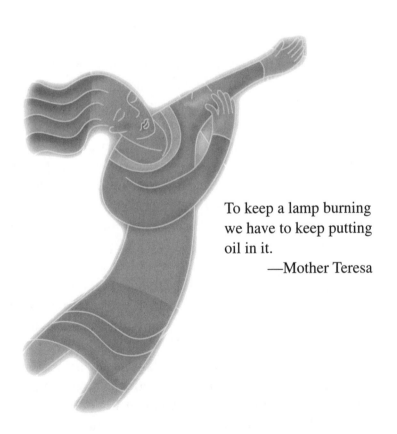

To keep a lamp burning
we have to keep putting
oil in it.
　　　—Mother Teresa

Your life's work is to exercise your mind, your spirit, and your body, so that you can realize your potential and enjoy being you. We ask you to stop, listen, and realize the ways your regular habits (life practices) are influencing your experiences. As a first step, simply try to think, feel, and act more optimistically. Listen to how you talk to (and about) yourself today and over the next few weeks. Look for common themes or patterns. Realizing what you are actually thinking and doing can lead you to make some meaningful changes, just as realizing that there is a pattern to your high blood sugar leads you to adjust your diabetes care habits.

## Life Practices

What practices do you use to manage your health and your diabetes? We call them practices because you are practicing ways to care for yourself. The ways you care for yourself change as you change. Practice is ongoing, not something that you achieve once and for all. It is a process of meeting your current needs by adding new practices or adapting them to whatever is going on in your life right now. Your health care team, support groups, and the information you gather can help you become aware of your needs and determine which practices to try. You are the one who determines which practices you adopt, whether they nurture you, and how to fit each one into your life. Adopting practices that are right for you is the first step toward wellness. You deserve the best, and you get to decide what the best is!

Okay, realizing what you need to do is one thing, but knowledge itself does not make the difference. Believing in yourself and changing your behavior does. You have already learned enough about healthy living to earn a PhD. Now is the time to commit the energy to practicing some of it. Make an investment in yourself.

It is common to begin a new practice and then to give up. New practices feel funny at first. Change is uncomfortable until it becomes habit. Generally, we either avoid the discomfort or try to do too many things at once and expect too much, too soon. As a result, we get frustrated and discouraged. Keep the following suggestions in mind as you adopt a new life practice.

1. Focus on one area of your life that you want to improve. To do this, you may need to stop, breathe, and reflect on what is important to you right now.
2. Visualize what is in this change for you. Identify the benefits you can expect from the new practice and remind yourself of them often.
3. Be practical. How? Allow yourself enough time to experiment and see the results. Pick one or two small practices to try. Stick with them for several weeks to a month.
4. Prioritize. Commit the time and other resources necessary to adopt the practice. Don't give up, be persistent. You are in training, just like an athlete.
5. Believe in yourself. Make the effort to help yourself. Show your commitment by telling yourself, "You can do it. You are worth the effort."
6. Expect challenges. Your energy and sense of commitment will go through peaks and valleys. Expect it. Your job is to prevent discouragement from affecting your ability to accomplish your goal. Seek assistance when you need it.
7. Enjoy your revitalized self. It is exhilarating to accomplish a goal. Enjoy the rewards of the new practice—a stronger, healthier, wiser you.
8. Build and use a support team to celebrate, and when necessary, motivate you.

Knowing what your health goals are provides the motivation to develop and maintain healthy life practices. These goals also help you get back on track when you are discouraged or bored. Everybody's goals are unique. Unless you set your own, they won't mean much to you. To help you identify what your goals are, think about what you would like to be doing in 5 years and then in 20 years.

Use the following list to help you identify your own goals. Be careful not to choose too many at one time.

Worthy personal goals are to
- improve managing my diabetes
- communicate my needs
- nurture an intimate relationship
- fulfill the needs once met by a relationship that has ended
- nurture my children
- prepare for a new venture (college, marriage, parenthood, retirement)
- initiate or nurture a friendship
- be fulfilled through volunteer work
- be fulfilled through my hobbies
- have fun
- simplify my lifestyle
- be fulfilled at work
- experience sensual pleasure
- enjoy companionship

Add your own goals. Now that you have identified an area or two in your life that you would like to improve, ask yourself what you need to do to achieve your goal. The things you choose to do will become the practices that help you achieve your vision for the future. For example, you can't change all the foods you eat in one day, but you can focus on trying to eat 5 servings of vegetables and fruit a day.

## How to Set Goals and Bring New Practices into Your Life

*Rudy is a 72-year-old woman with diabetes, heart disease, and kidney failure. She is legally blind and unable to walk great distances. She is disappointed that she cannot see the vibrant colors that she used to or walk where she would like. But it is her belief that this is God's message to her to use her brain more now.*

## *Take responsibility for yourself*

Say to yourself, "Even though I may resist at first, I accept that only by being responsible to myself can I fully express my talents and experience the gifts of my life."

**Establish yourself as a priority.** Before you can take responsibility for yourself, you need to promote yourself to the top of the priority list and give yourself the authority you need to take charge. Learn to say no. It is okay. Practice by taking over responsibilities for yourself in ways that you can manage right now. Learn to ask for assistance if you need it. It doesn't take away from your accomplishments or your commitment to others. Being "selfish" enough to take care of yourself and address your needs is healthy and a positive step toward wellness.

**Be realistic.** Make health goals that you can commit to doing. The keys are to

1. set a goal
2. define at least four steps you can take to reach it
3. determine realistic ways to take each step
4. commit to your plan
5. follow through
6. celebrate your successes
7. use mistakes to alter the plan to fit you better
8. appreciate each small step you take. Achieving success, no matter how small, and building on it will demonstrate your abilities and build your self-esteem.

**Communicate your needs.** Be aware of what others can and cannot give you. You manage your health practices. Then remember that they cannot read your mind. State your needs. Be an advocate for yourself as a woman and a person with diabetes. This might feel strange at first, especially if you are not accustomed to speaking about yourself. Speaking up for yourself is like lending support to a young child. There is no one more familiar with your personal needs and desires than you.

**Ask questions until the answers are clear to you.** Do the people in your life (at home, school, work, etc.) want the same things that you do? Do they know how to help you? How does your health care team look at diabetes? What health practices are they recommending? Why? How do they see you?

**Take calculated risks.** Try new things. Join a group. Take a course. Ask a question. When you fall, pick yourself up and try again. Begin to play again. Or if you never played as a child, it's time to learn how. Play hopscotch, jump rope. Go hang-gliding or horseback riding. Take up piano or violin lessons. Build a model airplane and fly it. Have some fun every day.

Say to yourself, "I respect the daily challenges that living with diabetes brings. I honor my own wisdom and accept my own limitations in meeting these challenges. Trusting in my own wisdom and the support of others, I can rise to meet these challenges and thrive."

**Find the help and information you need.** To live comfortably with diabetes, you need to learn as much as you can about diabetes and your body. This is a lifelong learning process. Getting the information you need and finding adequate support while you are learning can be both rewarding and challenging. Spending time with other women who are at similar places in their lives gives you information and support. People, publications, and the World Wide Web are all potential sources of useful support and information. You may feel pressured to learn everything all at once. Relax. You can only absorb so much at one time. Remember that emotions can cloud what you hear or read. Allow yourself to experience what is happening rather than forcing yourself to do things that you may not be ready for yet.

There are many wonderful diabetes programs and professionals to help you. Attending a diabetes education program is an important investment in your well-being. Even if your health insurance might not cover it, it is worth the money to learn the skills you need to live well with diabetes. The following is a list of diabetes self-care skills that you want to be sure you have. Do you need to seek additional training and support?

### Diabetes self-care skills
- Meal-planning strategies: how to plan your meals, count carbohydrates, read food labels, and make adjustments to the meal plan for unusual situations such as pregnancy or athletic events
- Activity guidelines: how to lead an active lifestyle and maintain body fitness
- Medication strategies: how and when to take medications, so they work best for you
- Monitoring: how to check blood glucose, interpret the readings, and respond to the numbers and patterns
- Hypoglycemia and hyperglycemia: how to detect, treat, and prevent them
- Sick-day management: how to prevent life-threatening problems, such as ketoacidosis
- Foot, skin, and dental care
- Screening for complications: the tests to have and the providers to see on a routine basis
- Guidelines for when to contact health care providers and who to contact
- Ways to reduce your individual risk factors for getting complications

## *Seeking the support of professionals*
You have the right to work with a team of professionals who listen and respond to your needs. Recognize and respect the limitations of your health care provider. Prepare for your visit, write down questions that will help your provider focus on and address your concerns, and identify the areas that make it difficult for you to take care of your diabetes. Help your doctor treat you as a per-

son. Report what is going on in your life that may be feeding (or draining) your energy and ability to follow your treatment program. Diabetes professionals want to provide you with valuable information. They are also there to help you be a problem-solver and figure out how to make the diabetes program work for you. It takes time, patience, and fine-tuning to find out what works. Don't give up. They are your partners, and they need your active participation.

## *Practice regular renewal*

Say to yourself, "I deserve the time and quiet to rejuvenate myself each day. Only in allowing myself to focus can I be whole, happy, and healthy."

You need practices to help you recover from the normal stresses of the day and to become more resilient for the bigger burdens you sometimes face. Stress, both physical and emotional, can be good for you as long as you have periods to recover. You recover when you relax and gather your energies to reflect on your experiences and grow. You may be uncomfortable investing time and energy in yourself, but this investment pays big dividends! As a human being, you rebuild and recover through sleep, eating good food, laughing, and spending time with yourself in a pleasant, focused way. Take the attitude of "I work hard, I play hard." Balance your energy. Be active. Be idle. They're both important.

Here are some practices you could adopt to relax from your daily stresses and renew yourself for jumping back into your life.

**Breathing.** Your best friend is your breath. It is always there. Conscious breathing is the most powerful way to focus, build your energy, and relax. All this is done simply by breathing deeply and rhythmically. You can practice this anywhere, at any time. With time and practice, you can develop the habit of responding to stressful situations with a calming breath instead of the more typical tightening up and shallow breathing. Practice getting in touch with your breathing by placing your hand on your belly. Breathe slowly (count of 8) into your belly, feeling it rise as you inhale.

Hold the breath far down in your abdomen for as long as you can. Let it out slowly and steadily for a count of 8. Relax and repeat. As you inhale, imagine bringing in warm air and sunshine. Exhale out any tension. Five minutes of abdominal breathing will give you lots of energy. Three such breaths in a tense situation can gather your forces quickly.

**Create pause in your life.** Slow down to listen to your body and replenish your energy stores. Get off the treadmill from time to time. In chapter 2, we speak about creating a vacation from some of your responsibilities. Discuss with a loved one or friend what others can do for or with you to give you some relief. There are things you can do for yourself. Being busy does not have to interfere with your ability to experience the moment. For example, if you are washing the dishes, instead of thinking about all of the other things you have to do, try to focus on the moment. Enjoy the warmth of the water, a sense of accomplishment as the clean dishes mount up, the weight of your body balanced on the balls of your feet, how you feel as you take slow, deep breaths. It is lovely to be alive in this moment; pay attention to it, and you'll have more energy for the next moment, too.

**Relaxation.** Relaxing is the art of doing what nurtures your body, slows down your mind, helps you ignore outside distractions, and focuses you inward. A hot bath, a nature walk, playing with your cat, reading, doing yoga, drinking a cup of tea, listening to music, taking a jog, or walking the dog are all ways that you can unwind and relax. Practicing meditation in any of its many forms calms your mind and body and lifts you into an elevated state of awareness. Achieving this state takes practice and commitment. You need to show up for your own renewal time each day. When you relax, you can be more aware of what is happening around you and inside you.

**Rest.** The average person requires 6 to 10 hours of sleep a night. Doing what you can to ensure a good night's rest gives you an edge on the day ahead. Nighttime hypoglycemia can really foul up your night and the next day. Work with your health care provider to resolve these sleep disturbances. Perhaps you need a snack at bedtime or to change your medication dosages. Sleep is a great and often overlooked healer.

When you are tired, rest. If you are tense, exercise, stretch, or do yoga to work the tension out of your body. Quiet your mind at the end of the day by relaxing with a hot bath, a good book, or meditation and set the stage for restful sleep. Make your resting place inviting and cozy. Watch your caffeine and alcohol intake before sleep. Think positive thoughts, and affirm your desire to gain perspective through sleep. Consciously clear your mind and relax your body. This daily practice is one of the most powerful ways to renew and rebuild your body and mind, yet little attention is paid to it. You perform best when you are relaxed and calm, when your energy is high, positive, and in control.

### *Take care of your body*

Say to yourself, "My body is amazing. By taking care of any single part of it, I am nurturing my entire body, mind, and spirit."

**Honoring your body as it is right now.** We are bombarded by messages to lose weight and fit into society's image of the ideal woman. If we focus on external images or measures, it is easy to think that something is wrong with our bodies. You honor your body through using it and listening to it. We must not accept the judgment of others to measure our own self-worth.

**Healthy eating.** Build a healthy relationship with food. You can lose or maintain weight when you exercise and eat sensibly. People who exercise as part of their weight-loss plan seldom gain back the weight they have lost. You are more likely to lose weight when you have muscle (it keeps on burning calories even at rest). Exercise helps you create muscle. When you diet, the first weight you lose is usually water. If you do not exercise, the next thing you lose is muscle. In addition, your metabolism slows down (as though you were going through a famine), and your body resists losing weight.

Food satisfies, rebuilds, energizes, and protects your body. It can also harm it. Your food choices and eating patterns influence your energy level, blood-glucose control, weight, and even your resistance and susceptibility to some forms of cancer and heart disease. Our culture of fast food and fad diets has led us away from eating for nutrition. This complicates eating for blood sugar control (and weight loss). You need to be sure you are getting the nutrients you need and that you enjoy and feel nourished by what you eat. See a dietitian who will work with you on these goals.

**Healthy skin.** Your skin is the largest organ in your body. It needs to be cleansed, moisturized, and nourished to maintain its beauty and ability to protect your body. Skin problems can be a sign of poor blood sugar control. If you have a skin problem, try to figure out why and treat the cause. Check your skin regularly. To keep your skin healthy regularly moisturize it with an oil-in-water cream, humidify your home, avoid long hot soaks in a bath or spa, treat cuts right away using antibiotic cream or ointment, eat healthfully, and drink plenty of water. Sodas, coffee, tea do not count as water. In fact, they remove water from your system.

**Body works.** It is important for you to get in touch with your body. The deep breathing and relaxation exercises described earlier is a place to start. Hands-on therapies such as massage, acupressure, or reflexology help you experience your body in new ways. In addition, give your body loving messages, and your body will respond in a positive way. Discard any critical messages. Andrew Weil in his book *Spontaneous Healing* suggests a practice for loving your body. First, identify one part of your body to work on, for instance, your belly. Second, stand in front of a mirror each day and focus on your belly. Speak to it directly, and tell it how much you love it. Tell it what you appreciate about it. "Belly, I love you. I appreciate that you hold my essence. Your shape is round and beautiful." Repeat statements such as these several times.

Continue focusing on this part of your body for several weeks. Then move on to another part of your body.

**Loosening up.** Stretching, yoga, massage, and laughter release the tensions that accumulate over the day. These techniques can increase your strength, flexibility, and endurance. A well-toned and flexible body is better able to respond to physical and emotional stresses. If your body feels happy, your mind feels better, too.

**Moving for recreation and fitness.** Put some more fun into your life. Get moving. Play! All children love to play. It is natural and a fun way to exercise. How you view what you do for movement can make the difference in whether you just endure it or truly enjoy it. Because your body, mind, and spirit are always connected, exercising your body will also invigorate the rest of you. You will improve your diabetes, reduce stress, get better quality sleep, improve the way your body uses food, enhance your self-image, and reduce your risk of heart disease. When you take the initiative to exercise, you make a statement of your personal power and desire to be in charge of your life. Sometimes this practice is difficult because of the pressure you put on yourself to do it right or to look just so. As a popular saying goes, "Dance as though no one is looking." Relax and move in ways that feel comfortable to you. Remember to keep your spine in good alignment by imagining a string going out of the top of your head pulling you up into an easy balanced posture. Now breathe!

> *Why aren't you dancing for joy at this very moment?*
>
> —Pir Vilayet Khan, Sufi seer

## Take care of your mind

Say to yourself, "I can gain mastery over my emotions and frustrations even though I may not be able to change the things that bother me. Clear thinking makes all of life's work easier."

**Keeping things straight.** Diabetes brings a lot of equipment and tasks into your life. Life presents unpredictable challenges. Keeping things straight can really cut down on the time and stress related to having diabetes. Practices that create order are liberating. You can make enough time to do the things you want while taking care of the things you must.

**Living in the present.** Focus on what you are doing right now. Give it your undivided attention. Make each moment count. You'll feel more connected and aware of the differences each day even in routine tasks.

**Simplifying.** Get rid of some of the tasks on your to-do list. Doing less while still meeting the challenges of life will give you more time to enjoy what life has to offer. Look at how you spend your time—keep a log if you need to—and consolidate or delete the things that are not necessary. Unclutter your life. Stop doing the things that you don't need or care about. Throw or give away things you don't use, such as clothes that don't fit. Plan several errands for one outing, like shopping for food when you go to get your hair cut or to the drug store. Whatever small steps you can take to simplify your life will bring you gifts of time and freedom.

**Organizing.** Make rituals for the things you do regularly. Keeping medication in the bathroom and taking it when you brush your teeth saves time and helps you remember to do it. Being organized means you have a place for things and take the responsibility to put them back. It also means that you have thought through what you will need and have it available when you are ready. It is impressive how many creative ways people with diabetes have discovered to carry food, insulin, medication, and blood-testing equipment with them. Being organized is an investment in your future. For some people, this comes naturally; for others, it requires quite a lot of discipline and practice.

**Quieting yourself.** Solitude—being alone with yourself—is very different from being lonely. The difference is how you treat yourself. If you listen, honor, and trust yourself, you will grow. This can sometimes be very uncomfortable. If you have ignored, shut out, and distanced yourself from your own feelings, tuning into them now will require patience and support. Quieting yourself is an art. There are many practices from hobbies to meditation that help you tune into yourself. These practices teach you ways to be calm and to put things into perspective.

**Practicing yoga, meditation, and tai chi.** These ancient practices provide a woman with the opportunity to tune into her body and quiet her mind at the same time. Deep breathing, centering, and stretching are key techniques used to focus the mind and body. Consider learning from someone who knows what they are doing, someone who can be a mentor as you make these new practices part of your routine.

**Being spontaneous.** Learn how to pack your bag, change your meal plan, or adjust your diabetes medication, so that you can be as spontaneous as possible and seize the opportunities that come your way.

**Gaining sustenance from doing what you love.** Fortunately, much of what women do is creative. This nourishes your heart and your spirit. Doing things that are creative and bring you gratification on a regular basis is one of the best ways to relax and relate to yourself. Gardening, ironing, cooking, dancing, reading, painting a picture, photographing nature, sewing, surfing the Net, or playing a musical instrument are all practices that can provide you with fulfillment. Many women find journal writing to be an effective means of connecting with their inner wisdom. Seek new ways to express who you are.

### Taking care of your spirit

Say to yourself, "I can connect with my own spirit by reaching out to others, reaching in to my beliefs, and befriending my enemies, real and imagined."

**Balancing your time and energy.** Balancing the time and energy you spend on meeting your responsibilities will lead to a more fulfilling life. Simply note how you divide your time between caring for yourself, caring for others, working, and playing. Distribute the time more evenly by focusing on the areas that get less of your attention right now.

**Scheduling time for you.** This may be the time when you plan your healthy meals, exercise, or meditate. Taking care of yourself requires time, so protect it. Do not give it up even for a loved one. Imagine there is a fence surrounding this time with a gate that only you can open. When you are asked to fit something else in, close the gate.

**Dealing with fear.** Fear, like anger, is a normal emotion, but it is difficult to vent and release. While anger stimulates you to run or fight, fear often paralyzes you or hides behind other emotions. Avoiding your instinct to be afraid is not a good idea, but controlling your response to it can be. Fears common to women are: fears of failure, of rejection, of the unknown, of dying or isolation, and of loss of self control. Do you know what you fear? Trying to avoid the things you fear may result in decisions that cause you and others pain. Facing what you fear, although difficult, is always better. It forces you to develop a strategy and find out more about your own power. Facing what you fear is tough! But when you do, it will pass. You will see how strong you are.

Fear is very closely related to your level of self-esteem. When you are down on yourself, you are more vulnerable and sensitive to the things you worry about and feeling afraid is common. Building up your self-esteem does a lot to allay fear.

**Allowing yourself to heal.** Let your tears flow. They can release emotions you can't express or recognize. Sit with the feelings. Try on different perspectives. Listen to the insights and new perspectives that rise from your intuition. Share your story. Write it down. Connect with a women's group. When you need to, seek the help of a professional who can provide an objective perspective and help you still the emotional chatter in your mind. Consider an attitude adjustment! Precious time and energy is lost being unhappy and focusing on things you cannot change. We need to focus on changing the things we can. Holding on to negative emotions is unhealthy.

**Creating more joy.** Laugh. Let the spunky five-year-old girl who lives inside of you come out to play. Giggle, be silly, squish jello between your fingers. Open yourself to experiencing life with the freedom and innocence of the little girl. Look more often through her eyes. Each moment is new. Each event is special.

**Befriending your enemies.** "An enemy is always a teacher in disguise," says every wisdom school in the world. An enemy makes you uncomfortable and challenges your life practices, your beliefs, and your worldview. An enemy makes you change and possibly grow. You may discover new beliefs about yourself, learn new things, and develop new ways to relate to the people around you. You may find that the practices you've been following are out of date. That's when you try on new ones and gradually replace the old ones to fit the person you want to be. Building on your new strengths and experience is the way to make changes that fit you. Work with, not against your own wisdom. Enemies can help you realize when you're fooling yourself.

**Affirming what you believe.** Affirmations are words you say to yourself throughout the day to reprogram how you view yourself and your life. This is positive self-talk. Just as an athlete develops muscle by practicing every day, they use affirmations that way, too. You can develop new beliefs about yourself and your abilities. Your mind and spirit are like muscles. To change a belief you need repetition, rehearsal, and practice, just as you do with building a muscle. You need to feed yourself with positive messages. Write down a short sentence that you can say to shift your thinking in the direction you want to go. For example, write "I communicate clearly" or "I am fun-loving." Write it on a piece of paper and put it where you will see it often. Read it several times each day, until it runs through your mind naturally. This practice helps make it easier to fit new practices, like meditation or exercise (play), into your life.

Here are more affirmations you can choose to repeat to yourself. Please create your own to fit your situation. You will soon see how positive statements of your own worth can be powerful tools to use.

- I am doing a great job!
- Boy, am I proud of the hard work I do to lose weight. Keep up the good work! I am amazing. I handle so much and balance so many things in my life that most women don't even think about once in their lives.
- I do a great job juggling the house, kids, school, and work.
- I love me for trying.
- I am a wonderful and capable person.
- I can make life decisions and be happy with them.
- I admire my strength in this new part of my life.
- I'm a great mom!
- My hard work has made a difference.
- I take care of my diabetes as well as I can.
- I make a refreshing difference in other people's lives.
- I forgive myself.
- My sense of humor is refreshing.
- When I am not in great control, I am not bad or wrong in my care techniques.
- I am okay just the way I am!
- All qualities exist in me. In each moment, I can choose the one I need.
- I am beautiful.

Each of us needs to remember the wisdom of our youth.

*I think I am very attractive. Who doesn't? Everyone is attractive, no matter what they look like. It's what is on the inside that counts, not on the outside. It's also your personality. I think that I am very unique and that is what makes me so special.*

—Siobhan Perkins (age 12)

# Recommended Reading

*A Woman's Worth*. Marianne Williamson, Ballantine Books, New York, 1994.

*Women Who Run With the Wolves*. Clarissa Pinkola Estés, PhD, Ballantine Books, New York, 1992.

*A Woman's Journey to God*. Joan Borysenko, MD, Riverhead Books, New York, 1999.

*The Woman's Book of Courage: Meditations for Empowerment and Peace of Mind*. Sue Patton Thoele, Conari Press, Berkeley, California, 1991.

*Simple Abundance*. Sarah Ban Breathnach, Time Warner, New York, 1995.

*The Path of Love*. Deepak Chopra, Harmony Books, New York, 1997.

*Anatomy of the Spirit*. Caroline Myss, Harmony Books, New York, 1996. (audio tapes)

*Spiritual Literacy: Reading the Sacred in Everyday Life*. Frederic and Mary Ann Brussat, Scribner, New York, 1996.

*The Women We Become*. Ann Thomas, Prima Publishing, Rocklin, California, 1997.

*The Art of the Possible*. Alexandra Stoddard, Avon Books, New York, 1995.

*NeuroSpeak*. Robert Masters, Quest Books, Wheaton, Illinois, 1994.

# Index

# About the American Diabetes Association

The American Diabetes Association is the nation's leading voluntary health organization supporting diabetes research, information, and advocacy. Its mission is to prevent and cure diabetes and to improve the lives of all people affected by diabetes. The American Diabetes Association is the leading publisher of comprehensive diabetes information. Its huge library of practical and authoritative books for people with diabetes covers every aspect of self-care—cooking and nutrition, fitness, weight control, medications, complications, emotional issues, and general self-care.

**To order American Diabetes Association books:** Call 1-800-232-6733. http://store.diabetes.org [Note: there is no need to use **www** when typing this particular Web address]

**To join the American Diabetes Association:** Call 1-800-806-7801. www.diabetes.org/membership

**For more information about diabetes or ADA programs and services:** Call 1-800-342-2383. E-mail: Customerservice@diabetes.org www.diabetes.org

**To locate an ADA/NCQA Recognized Provider of quality diabetes care in your area:** Call 1-703-549-1500 ext. 2202. www.diabetes.org/recognition/Physicians/ListAll.asp

**To find an ADA Recognized Education Program in your area:** Call 1-888-232-0822. www.diabetes.org/recognition/education.asp

**To join the fight to increase funding for diabetes research, end discrimination, and improve insurance coverage:** Call 1-800-342-2383. www.diabetes.org/advocacy

**To find out how you can get involved with the programs in your community:** Call 1-800-342-2383. See below for program Web addresses.

- *American Diabetes Month:* Educational activities aimed at those diagnosed with diabetes—month of November. www.diabetes.org/ADM
- *American Diabetes Alert:* Annual public awareness campaign to find the undiagnosed—held the fourth Tuesday in March. www.diabetes.org/alert
- *The Diabetes Assistance & Resources Program (DAR):* diabetes awareness program targeted to the Latino community. www.diabetes.org/DAR
- *African American Program:* diabetes awareness program targeted to the African American community. www.diabetes.org/africanamerican
- *Awakening the Spirit: Pathways to Diabetes Prevention & Control:* diabetes awareness program targeted to the Native American community. www.diabetes.org/awakening

**To find out about an important research project regarding type 2 diabetes:** www.diabetes.org/ada/research.asp

**To obtain information on making a planned gift or charitable bequest:** Call 1-888-700-7029. www.diabetes.org/ada/plan.asp

**To make a donation or memorial contribution:** Call 1-800-342-2383. www.diabetes.org/ada/cont.asp